LOUISA CRONIN

BLOOD TYPE A'S

COOKBOOK FOR VEGETARIANS

DELICIOUS AND NUTRITIOUS PLANT-BASED RECIPES TO NOURISH AND THRIVE

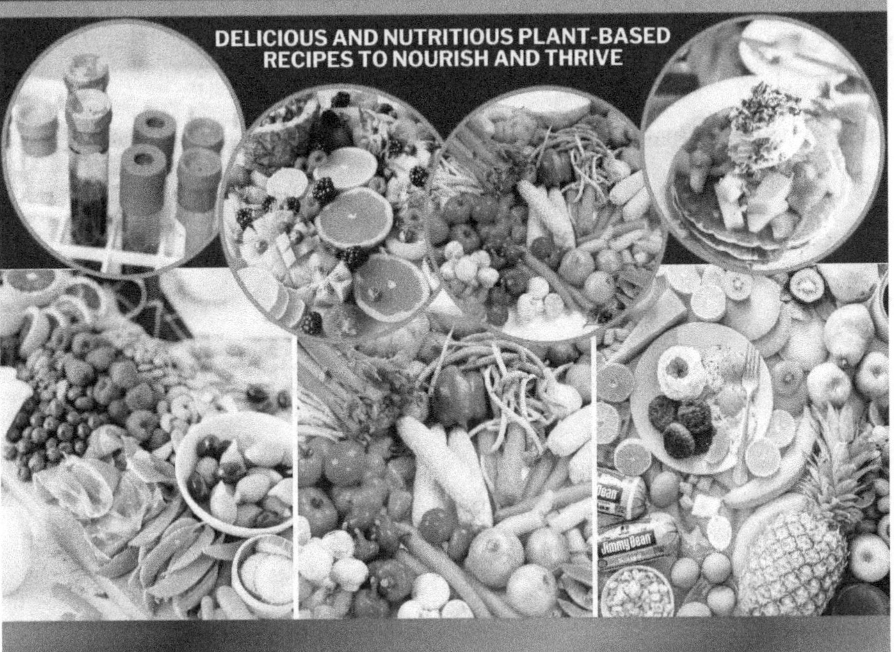

COPYRIGHTS

DEDICATION

To anyone who seeks delicious and healthy vegetarian meals. May this book spark your creativity in the kitchen and fill your life with vibrant plant-based dishes!

Table of Contents

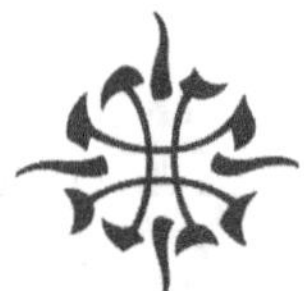

Chapter 1

Introduction to Blood Type A Diet

Understanding the Blood Type A Diet

The Blood Type A Diet is a dietary approach that focuses on the unique nutritional needs of individuals with blood type A. Developed by naturopathic physician Dr. Peter J. D'Adamo, the diet suggests that people with blood type A can optimize their health and prevent certain diseases by following a specific eating plan tailored to their blood type.

According to the Blood Type A Diet, individuals with blood type A are believed to have evolved from agrarian ancestors who primarily consumed plant-based foods. As a result, this diet emphasizes a vegetarian or vegan approach, with a focus on fresh fruits, vegetables, whole grains, legumes, and soy-based products. It recommends limiting or avoiding animal protein, particularly red meat and dairy products.

The rationale behind the Blood Type A Diet lies in the concept that certain lectins, which are proteins found in foods, can react differently with each blood type. Dr. D'Adamo suggests that lectins in certain foods can agglutinate, or clump together, with blood cells of specific blood types, leading to various health issues. Therefore, he recommends avoiding the lectins that may be problematic for individuals with blood type A.

In addition to the emphasis on plant-based foods, the Blood Type A Diet also encourages regular physical activity, stress reduction techniques such as yoga or meditation, and adequate sleep. These lifestyle factors are believed to complement the dietary guidelines and promote overall well-being for individuals with blood type A.

While the Blood Type A Diet has gained popularity, it's essential to note that scientific evidence supporting its claims is limited. The concept of blood type diets is controversial within the scientific community, and more research is needed to validate the specific dietary recommendations for each blood type. However, some individuals may find that following this eating plan aligns with their personal preferences and leads to positive health outcomes.

BENEFITS OF A VEGETARIAN LIFESTYLE

A vegetarian lifestyle involves abstaining from the consumption of meat, poultry, and seafood, while still including plant-based foods such as fruits, vegetables, grains, legumes, nuts, and seeds. Many people choose to adopt a vegetarian diet for various reasons, including health, environmental concerns, animal welfare, or personal beliefs. There are several potential benefits associated with following a vegetarian lifestyle.

One of the primary advantages of a vegetarian diet is its potential to promote overall health and reduce the risk of chronic diseases. Plant-based diets are typically rich in fiber, vitamins, minerals, and phytochemicals, which are beneficial compounds naturally found in plants. These nutrients are essential for maintaining optimal health and reducing the risk of conditions such as heart disease, obesity, type 2 diabetes, and certain types of cancer.

Studies have shown that vegetarians often have lower body mass indexes (BMIs) and reduced rates of obesity compared to their meat-eating counterparts. Plant-based diets tend to be lower in calories and saturated fats while being higher in fiber, which can contribute to weight management and improved metabolic health.

Furthermore, vegetarian diets can be a valuable tool in reducing environmental impact. Animal agriculture has been linked to deforestation, water pollution, greenhouse gas emissions, and other environmental concerns. By choosing a vegetarian lifestyle, individuals can help decrease their ecological footprint and contribute to a more sustainable planet.

Adopting a vegetarian lifestyle can also promote animal welfare by reducing the demand for meat and animal products. It aligns with the belief that animals should be treated with compassion and respect, and many individuals find ethical satisfaction in not supporting industries that involve animal exploitation.

It's important to note that while a vegetarian diet can provide numerous health benefits, it requires careful planning to ensure adequate intake of essential nutrients such as protein, iron, vitamin B12, and omega-3 fatty acids. Vegetarians should be mindful of incorporating a variety of plant-based protein sources, fortified foods, and, if necessary, appropriate supplements to meet their nutritional needs.

TIPS FOR SUCCESSFUL MEAL PLANNING

Meal planning is a valuable tool for individuals seeking to maintain a healthy and well-balanced diet. Planning meals in advance helps save time, reduce stress, and ensure that nutritious options are readily available. Whether you're following a specific diet or simply aiming to make healthier choices, here are some tips for successful meal planning.

1. Set aside dedicated time: Allocate a specific time each week to plan your meals. This can be a few hours on the weekend or any other convenient time. Having a designated time ensures that you prioritize meal planning and make it a regular part of your routine.

2. Consider your schedule and preferences: Take into account your daily activities, work schedule, and personal preferences when planning meals. Consider the number of meals you need to prepare, whether you require portable options, and any dietary restrictions or food allergies.

3. Create a menu: Start by creating a menu for the week or a set number of days. Include a variety of foods from different food groups to ensure a balanced diet. Consider incorporating seasonal ingredients to add freshness and flavor to your meals.

4. Make a shopping list: Once you have your menu, create a comprehensive shoppinglist based on the ingredients needed for your planned meals. Having a well-organized shopping list ensures that you don't forget any essential items and helps you avoid impulse purchases.

5. Shop with intention: When you go grocery shopping, stick to your list and avoid unnecessary temptations. Focus on the perimeter of the store, where fresh produce, whole grains, and lean proteins are typically located. Minimize the amount of processed and unhealthy foods you bring home.

6. Prep ahead of time: Take advantage of any free time you have to pre-prep ingredients or even whole meals. Chop vegetables, marinate proteins, or cook grains in advance, so you have them ready to use during busy weekdays. This can significantly reduce meal preparation time and make it easier to stick to your planned meals.

7. Embrace batch cooking: Consider batch cooking large quantities of staple foods such as grains, legumes, or sauces. You can portion them out and freeze them for later use. This approach saves time and ensures that you always have healthy options available, especially on days when you're short on time or energy.

8. Use leftovers creatively: Don't let leftovers go to waste. Get creative and repurpose them into new meals. For example, leftover roasted vegetables can be added to salads or turned into a delicious omelet the next day. This not only saves time but also adds variety to your meals.

9. Stay flexible: Meal planning is meant to be a helpful guide, but it's okay to deviate from it occasionally. Life happens, and unexpected events or changing preferences may arise. Adapt your plan as needed and make adjustments to accommodate any changes that come up.

10. Enjoy the process: Meal planning doesn't have to be a chore. Embrace it as an opportunity to explore new recipes,

try different flavors, and nourish your body. Involve family members or roommates in the planning process to make it a collaborative and enjoyable experience.

Remember, successful meal planning is about finding a system that works for you. Experiment with different approaches and strategies until you find what suits your lifestyle and dietary goals. With consistency and a little bit of effort, meal planning can contribute to healthier eating habits and make your daily meals more enjoyable and stress-free.

ESSENTIAL NUTRIENTS FOR BLOOD TYPE A

While the Blood Type A Diet focuses on specific dietary recommendations for individuals with blood type A, it's important to note that the concept of blood type diets lacks scientific evidence. However, if you choose to follow this dietary approach, it's essential to ensure you're getting all the necessary nutrients to support your overall health. Here are some essential nutrients to consider when following the Blood Type A Diet:

1. Protein: Since the Blood Type A Diet recommends limiting or avoiding animal protein, it's important to find alternative sources of protein. Good plant-based protein options for blood type A individuals include soy products (such as tofu

and tempeh), legumes (such as lentils, chickpeas, and kidney beans), quinoa, and certain nuts and seeds.

2. Calcium: Since dairy products are limited on the Blood Type A Diet, it's important to find other sources of calcium. Good plant-based sources of calcium include dark leafy greens (such as kale and broccoli), almonds, sesame seeds, and fortified plant-based milk alternatives (such as almond milk or soy milk).

3. Iron: Iron is essential for carrying oxygen in the blood. While plant-based sources of iron are abundant, it's important to note that the iron from plant-based foods is less readily absorbed than the iron from animal sources. Good plant-based sources of iron for blood type A individuals include spinach, lentils, tofu, quinoa, and pumpkin seeds. Consuming vitamin C-rich foods, such as citrus fruits or bell peppers, alongside iron-rich foods can help enhance iron absorption.

4. Vitamin B12: Vitamin B12 is primarily found in animal-based foods, so individuals following a vegetarian or vegan diet, as recommended for blood type A, should consider supplementation or consuming fortified foods. Fortified plant-based milk alternatives, nutritional yeast, and certain plant-based meat substitutes may contain vitamin B12.

5. Omega-3 fatty acids: Omega-3 fatty acids play a crucial role in heart health and brain function. Good plant-based sources of omega-3s for blood type A individuals include flaxseeds, chia seeds, walnuts, and algae-based supplements.

It's important to emphasize that if you decide to follow the Blood Type A Diet or any specific dietary approach, it's advisable to consult with a registered dietitian or healthcare professional to ensure you're meeting your individual nutritional needs.

INCORPORATING EXERCISE AND MINDFULNESS

In addition to dietary considerations, incorporating exercise and mindfulness practices can further support your overall well-being, regardless of your blood type. Here are some tips for incorporating exercise and mindfulness into your routine:

1. Exercise:

- Find activities you enjoy: Choose physical activities that you genuinely enjoy, whether it's going for a walk, cycling, dancing, practicing yoga, or playing a sport. When you enjoy the exercise, you're more likely to stick with it.

- Set realistic goals: Start with small, achievable goals and gradually increase the intensity or duration of your workouts.

This approach helps prevent burnout or injury and allows for steady progress over time.

- Mix it up: Incorporate a variety of exercises to keep your routine interesting and to work different muscle groups. This can include cardiovascular exercises, strength training, flexibility exercises, and balance activities.

- Schedule regular exercise: Make exercise a priority by scheduling it into your daily or weekly routine. Treat it as an important appointment with yourself.

- Be mindful of your body: Listen to your body and adjust your exercise routine accordingly. Pay attention to any discomfort or pain and modify or seek professional advice if necessary.

2. Mindfulness:

- Practice meditation: Set aside a few minutes each day for meditation or mindfulness exercises. Focus on your breath, observe your thoughts without judgment, and cultivate a sense of presence and awareness.

- Engage in mindful eating: Pay attention to your food choices, eating habits, and the sensations of taste, smell, and texture while eating. Eat slowly, savor each bite, and try to be fully present during meals.

- Find moments of stillness: Take short breaks throughout the day to pause, breathe, and center yourself. This can be as simple as taking a few deep breaths or stepping outside for a short walk in nature.

- Connect with nature: Spend time in nature and appreciate the beauty around you. Engaging with natural environments can help reduce stress and promote a sense of calm and well-being.

- Practice gratitude: Cultivate a sense of gratitude by reflecting on the positive aspects of your life. This can be done through journaling or simply taking a few moments each day to express gratitude for the things you appreciate.

Incorporating exercise and mindfulness into your lifestyle can have numerous benefits, including stress reduction, improved mood, increased focus, enhanced physical fitness, and overall well-being. Find activities and practices that resonate with you and make them a regular part of your routine. Remember, consistency is key, and small steps can lead to significant positive changesPlease note that while the information provided above is based on general knowledge and recommendations, it's always advisable to consult with a healthcare professional, registered dietitian, or fitness instructor for personalized advice, especially if you have specific health concerns or conditions.

Chapter 2

Salads & Appetizers

Here are the recipes for the refreshing watermelon salad, Mediterranean quinoa salad, caprese skewers with balsamic glaze, Greek salad with tofu feta, and spinach and strawberry salad:

REFRESHING WATERMELON SALAD:

Preparation time: 15 minutes

Servings: 4

Ingredients:

- 4 cups cubed watermelon

- 1 cup sliced cucumber

- 1/2 cup crumbled feta cheese

- 1/4 cup chopped fresh mint leaves

- 2 tablespoons lime juice

- Salt and pepper to taste

Directions:

1. In a large bowl, combine the watermelon, cucumber, feta cheese, and mint leaves.

2. Drizzle the lime juice over the salad and gently toss to combine.

3. Season with salt and pepper to taste.

4. Serve chilled.

Nutrition (per serving):

Calories: 96

Carbohydrates: 13g

Protein: 4g

Fat: 4g

Fiber: 1g

MEDITERRANEAN QUINOA SALAD:

Preparation time: 20 minutes

Cooking time: 15 minutes

Servings: 4

Ingredients:

- 1 cup cooked quinoa

- 1 cup diced cucumber

- 1 cup cherry tomatoes, halved

- 1/2 cup diced red onion

- 1/4 cup chopped Kalamata olives

- 1/4 cup crumbled feta cheese

- 2 tablespoons chopped fresh parsley

- 2 tablespoons lemon juice

- 1 tablespoon extra-virgin olive oil

- Salt and pepper to taste

Directions:

1. In a large bowl, combine the cooked quinoa, cucumber, cherry tomatoes, red onion, Kalamata olives, feta cheese, and parsley.

2. In a small bowl, whisk together the lemon juice, olive oil, salt, and pepper.

3. Pour the dressing over the quinoa mixture and toss to combine.

4. Serve at room temperature or chilled.

Nutrition (per serving):

Calories: 198

Carbohydrates: 26g

Protein: 7g

Fat: 8g

Fiber: 4g

Caprese Skewers with Balsamic Glaze:

Preparation time: 10 minutes

Servings: 4

Ingredients:

- 1 pint cherry tomatoes

- 8 ounces fresh mozzarella cheese, cut into bite-sized pieces

- Fresh basil leaves

- Balsamic glaze for drizzling

- Salt and pepper to taste

Directions:

1. Thread a cherry tomato, a piece of mozzarella cheese, and a basil leaf onto a skewer.

2. Repeat the process until all the ingredients are used.

3. Arrange the skewers on a platter.

4. Drizzle with balsamic glaze and season with salt and pepper.

5. Serve immediately.

Nutrition (per serving):

Calories: 142

Carbohydrates: 5g

Protein: 11g

Fat: 9g

Fiber: 1g

GREEK SALAD WITH TOFU FETA:

Preparation time: 15 minutes

Servings: 4

Ingredients:

- 4 cups chopped romaine lettuce

- 1 cup cherry tomatoes, halved

- 1/2 cup cucumber, diced

- 1/4 cup sliced red onion

- 1/4 cup sliced Kalamata olives

- 1/4 cup crumbled tofu feta cheese (or regular feta cheese if not vegan)

- 2 tablespoons extra-virgin olive oil

- 1 tablespoon red wine vinegar

- 1 teaspoon dried oregano

- Salt and pepper to taste

Directions:

1. In a large bowl, combine the romaine lettuce, cherry tomatoes, cucumber, red onion, Kalamata olives, and tofu feta cheese.

2. In a small bowl, whisk together the olive oil, red wine vinegar, dried oregano, salt, and pepper.

3. Pour the dressing over the salad and toss to coat evenly.

4. Serve immediately.

Nutrition (per serving):

Calories: 111

Carbohydrates: 7g

Protein: 3g

Fat: 9g

Fiber: 2g

SPINACH AND STRAWBERRY SALAD:

Preparation time: 10 minutes

Servings: 4

Ingredients:

- 4 cups baby spinach leaves

- 1 cup sliced strawberries

- 1/4 cup crumbled goat cheese (or dairy-free cheese if preferred)

- 2 tablespoons sliced almonds

- 2 tablespoons balsamic vinaigrette dressing

- Salt and pepper to taste

Directions:

1. In a large bowl, combinethe baby spinach, sliced strawberries, crumbled goat cheese, and sliced almonds.

2. Drizzle the balsamic vinaigrette dressing over the salad and toss to coat evenly.

3. Season with salt and pepper to taste.

4. Serve immediately.

Nutrition (per serving):

Calories: 92

Carbohydrates: 6g

Protein: 4g

Fat: 6g

Fiber: 2g

Please note that the nutrition information provided is approximate and may vary depending on the specific ingredients and brands used.

Avocado Bruschetta:

Preparation time: 15 minutes

Cooking time: 5 minutes

Servings: 4

Ingredients:

- 4 slices of whole-grain bread

- 2 ripe avocados

- 1 small tomato, diced

- 1 clove of garlic, minced

- 1 tablespoon of fresh lemon juice

- 2 tablespoons of chopped fresh basil

- Salt and pepper to taste

Directions:

1. Toast the slices of whole-grain bread until golden brown.

2. In a bowl, mash the ripe avocados with a fork until smooth.

3. Add the diced tomato, minced garlic, fresh lemon juice, chopped basil, salt, and pepper to the mashed avocados. Mix well.

4. Spread the avocado mixture evenly on top of each toasted bread slice.

5. Garnish with additional chopped basil, if desired.

6. Serve the avocado bruschetta as a delicious appetizer or a light snack.

Nutrition:

Avocado bruschetta is a nutritious and flavorful dish. Avocados are rich in healthy fats, fiber, and various vitamins and minerals. They provide a creamy texture and a good source of monounsaturated fats, which are beneficial for heart health. The addition of tomatoes adds a dose of vitamin C and antioxidants, while fresh basil contributes to the overall taste and offers potential anti-inflammatory properties. Enjoy this tasty bruschetta while benefiting from the goodness of its ingredients.

ROASTED BEET HUMMUS:

Preparation time: 10 minutes

Cooking time: 45 minutes

Servings: 6

Ingredients:

- 2 medium-sized beets, roasted and peeled

- 1 can (15 ounces) of chickpeas, drained and rinsed

- 2 cloves of garlic

- 2 tablespoons of tahini

- 2 tablespoons of fresh lemon juice

- 2 tablespoons of extra-virgin olive oil

- Salt and pepper to taste

- Optional toppings: chopped fresh parsley, toasted sesame seeds

Directions:

1. Preheat the oven to 400°F (200°C). Wrap the beets in aluminum foil and roast them for about 45 minutes, or until they are tender when pierced with a fork. Let them cool, then peel and chop into smaller pieces.

2. In a food processor or blender, combine the roasted beets, chickpeas, garlic, tahini, fresh lemon juice, extra-virgin olive oil, salt, and pepper. Blend until smooth and creamy.

3. If the hummus is too thick, add a splash of water or additional olive oil to achieve the desired consistency.

4. Transfer the roasted beet hummus to a serving bowl and garnish with chopped fresh parsley and toasted sesame seeds, if desired.

5. Serve with pita bread, vegetable sticks, or your favorite crackers.

Nutrition:

Roasted beet hummus is not only visually appealing with its vibrant pink color, but it also offers a range of nutritional benefits. Beets are a great source of fiber, folate, and potassium, and they contain antioxidants that may help reduce inflammation and support heart health. Chickpeas provide protein, dietary fiber, and important minerals such as iron and magnesium. The addition of tahini, made from sesame seeds, contributes healthy fats and adds a distinct nutty flavor. Enjoy this delicious and nutritious hummus as a dip or spread for a satisfying snack or appetizer.

Cucumber and Tomato Salsa:

Preparation time: 10 minutes

Servings: 4

Ingredients:

- 1 large cucumber, diced

- 2 ripe tomatoes, diced

- 1/4 red onion, finely chopped

- 1 jalapeno pepper, seeded and finely chopped

- 2 tablespoons of fresh lime juice

- 1 tablespoon of chopped fresh cilantro

- Salt and pepper to taste

Directions:

1. In a bowl, combine the diced cucumber, diced tomatoes, finely chopped red onion, and finely chopped jalapeno pepper.

2. Add the fresh lime juice and chopped cilantro to the bowl. Mix well.

3. Season with salt and pepper according to your taste preferences.

4. Let the cucumber and tomato salsa sit for a few minutes to allow the flavors to meld together.

5. Serve as a refreshing and tangy accompaniment to grilled vegetables, tacos, or tortilla chips.

Nutrition:

Cucumber and tomato salsa is a light and refreshing dish that provides a burst of flavors. Cucumbers are hydrating and low in calories, while tomatoes offer a good amount of vitamin C, antioxidants, and lycopene, known for its potential health benefits. Red onions and jalapeno peppers add a mild heat and contribute additional antioxidants and phytonutrients.

Lime juice adds a zesty tang and provides a dose of vitamin C. This salsa is a great way to incorporate more vegetables into your diet while enjoying a delicious and nutritious condiment.

Zucchini Fritters with Yogurt Sauce:

Preparation time: 20 minutes

Cooking time: 15 minutes

Servings: 4

Ingredients:

- 2 medium zucchinis, grated

- 1/2 teaspoon of salt

- 1/4 cup of all-purpose flour

- 1/4 cup of grated Parmesan cheese

- 1 clove of garlic, minced

- 1/4 teaspoon of dried oregano

- 1/4 teaspoon of dried basil

- 1/4 teaspoon of black pepper

- 2 tablespoons of olive oil (for frying)

Yogurt Sauce:

- 1/2 cup of plain Greek yogurt

- 1 tablespoon of fresh lemon juice

- 1 tablespoon of chopped fresh dill

- Salt and pepper to taste

Directions:

1. Place the grated zucchinis in a colander and sprinkle with salt. Let them sit for about 10 minutes to allow excess moisture to drain. Squeeze out any remaining liquid using a clean kitchen towel or paper towels.

2. In a large bowl, combine the grated zucchinis, all-purpose flour, grated Parmesan cheese, minced garlic, dried oregano, dried basil, and black pepper. Mix well until all the ingredients are evenly incorporated.

3. Heat olive oil in a skillet over medium heat. Take a spoonful of the zucchini mixture and flatten it to form a small fritter. Place it in the skillet and repeat with the remaining mixture, making sure not to overcrowd the pan.

4. Cook the fritters for about 3-4 minutes on each side, or until they are golden brown and crispy. Remove them from the skillet and place them on a paper towel-lined plate to absorb any excess oil.

5. In a small bowl, whisk together the plain Greek yogurt, fresh lemon juice, chopped fresh dill, salt, and pepper to make the yogurt sauce.

6. Serve the zucchini fritters hot, with a dollop of yogurt sauce on top. They make a fantastic appetizer or a light main course.

Nutrition:

Zucchini fritters are a delightful way to enjoy the versatility and health benefits of this nutritious vegetable. Zucchinis are low in calories and high in fiber, vitamins A and C, and minerals such as potassium and manganese. The addition of Parmesan cheese provides a savory flavor and a boost of calcium. These fritters are pan-fried with minimal oil, making them a healthier alternative to deep-fried options. Paired with the tangy yogurt sauce, these zucchini fritters offer a satisfying combination of flavors and textures that will leave you feeling nourished and satisfied.

Quinoa Stuffed Mushrooms:

Preparation time: 15 minutes

Cooking time: 25 minutes

Servings: 4

Ingredients:

- 8 large white button mushrooms

- 1 cup of cooked quinoa

- 1/4 cup of diced red bell pepper

- 1/4 cup of diced zucchini

- 1/4 cup of diced onion

- 1 clove of garlic, minced

- 2 tablespoons of olive oil

- 1/4 teaspoon of dried thyme

- 1/4 teaspoon of dried rosemary

- Salt and pepper to taste

- Optional toppings: grated Parmesan cheese, chopped fresh parsley

Directions:

1. Preheat the oven to 375°F (190°C). Remove the stems from the mushrooms and set them aside. Place the mushroom caps on a baking sheet lined with parchment paper.

2. Finely chop the reserved mushroom stems.

3. In a skillet, heat olive oil over medium heat. Add the chopped mushroom stems, diced red bell pepper, diced

zucchini, diced onion, and minced garlic. Sauté until the vegetables are tender.

4. In a bowl, combine the cooked quinoa, sautéed vegetable mixture, dried thyme, dried rosemary, salt, and pepper. Mix well.

5. Spoon the quinoa mixture into each mushroom cap, filling them generously.

6. Bake the stuffed mushrooms in the preheated oven for about 20-25 minutes, or until the mushrooms are tender and the filling is heated through.

7. If desired, sprinkle grated Parmesan cheese and chopped fresh parsley on top of the stuffed mushrooms before serving.

8. Enjoy these quinoa stuffed mushrooms as a delightful appetizer or as a satisfying side dish.

Nutrition:

Quinoa stuffed mushrooms offer a combination of earthy flavors and wholesome ingredients. Mushrooms are low in calories and rich in vitamins and minerals, including B vitamins, selenium, and potassium. Quinoa, a complete protein, provides essential amino acids and is a good source of fiber. The addition of vegetables like red bell pepper, zucchini, and onion adds a variety of vitamins, minerals, and antioxidants to the dish. This recipe is a nutritious and flavorful way to enjoy

Sweet Potato and Black Bean Quesadillas:

Preparation time: 15 minutes

Cooking time: 20 minutes

Servings: 4

Ingredients:

- 2 medium sweet potatoes, peeled and diced

- 1 can (15 ounces) of black beans, drained and rinsed

- 1 small red onion, diced

- 2 cloves of garlic, minced

- 1 teaspoon of ground cumin

- 1/2 teaspoon of chili powder

- Salt and pepper to taste

- 4 large flour tortillas

- 1 cup of shredded cheddar cheese

- Optional toppings: salsa, guacamole, sour cream

Directions:

1. Place the diced sweet potatoes in a microwave-safe bowl and cook them in the microwave for about 5 minutes, or until they are tender. Alternatively, you can steam or boil the sweet potatoes until tender.

2. In a skillet, heat some oil over medium heat. Add the diced red onion and minced garlic. Sauté until the onion is translucent and fragrant.

3. Add the cooked sweet potatoes, black beans, ground cumin, chili powder, salt, and pepper to the skillet. Stir well to combine and cook for an additional 2-3 minutes, allowing the flavors to meld.

4. Lay out one flour tortilla and spread a quarter of the sweet potato and black bean mixture on one half of the tortilla.

5. Sprinkle a quarter of the shredded cheddar cheese over the sweet potato and black bean mixture.

6. Fold the tortilla in half, pressing gently to seal.

7. Repeat the process with the remaining tortillas and filling.

8. In a clean skillet, heat some oil over medium heat. Cook each quesadilla for 2-3 minutes on each side, or until they are golden brown and the cheese is melted.

9. Cut the quesadillas into wedges and serve hot with salsa, guacamole, and sour cream, if desired.

Nutrition:

Sweet potato and black bean quesadillas are a tasty and satisfying option packed with nutrients. Sweet potatoes are a great source of vitamins A and C, fiber, and antioxidants. Black beans provide protein, fiber, and various minerals, including iron and folate. The combination of these ingredients offers a balance of carbohydrates, protein, and healthy fats. Enjoy these quesadillas as a delicious and filling meal.

LENTIL AND VEGETABLE SOUP:

Preparation time: 15 minutes

Cooking time: 30 minutes

Servings: 6

Ingredients:

- 1 cup of dried lentils, rinsed and drained

- 1 tablespoon of olive oil

- 1 onion, diced

- 2 carrots, diced

- 2 celery stalks, diced

- 3 cloves of garlic, minced

- 1 can (14 ounces) of diced tomatoes

- 4 cups of vegetable broth

- 2 cups of water

- 1 teaspoon of dried thyme

- 1 teaspoon of dried oregano

- Salt and pepper to taste

- Fresh parsley for garnish (optional)

Directions:

1. In a large pot, heat the olive oil over medium heat. Add the diced onion, carrots, celery, and minced garlic. Sauté until the vegetables are softened.

2. Add the rinsed lentils, diced tomatoes (including the juice), vegetable broth, water, dried thyme, dried oregano, salt, and pepper to the pot. Stir well to combine.

3. Bring the soup to a boil, then reduce the heat to low. Cover the pot and simmer for about 25-30 minutes, or until the lentils are tender.

4. Taste the soup and adjust the seasoning if needed.

5. Ladle the lentil and vegetable soup into bowls and garnish with fresh parsley, if desired.

6. Serve the soup hot as a comforting and nutritious meal.

Nutrition:

Lentil and vegetable soup is a hearty and nourishing dish that provides a good amount of plant-based protein, fiber, and essential nutrients. Lentils are a great source of protein, iron, and folate, while vegetables like carrots, celery, and onions offer vitamins, minerals, and antioxidants. The combination of these ingredients creates a flavorful and satisfying soup that is also low in fat and cholesterol. Enjoy this wholesome soup as a nutritious lunch or dinner option.

STUFFED BELL PEPPERS WITH COUSCOUS:

Preparation time: 20 minutes

Cooking time: 45 minutes

Servings: 4

Ingredients:

- 4 large bell peppers (any color), tops removed and seeded

- 1 cup of cooked couscous

- 1 small onion, diced

- 2 cloves of garlic, minced

- 1 zucchini, diced

- 1 carrot, diced

- 1 can (14 ounces) of diced tomatoes

- 1/2 cup of grated mozzarella cheese

- 1/4 cup of chopped fresh parsley

- 2 tablespoons of olive oil

- 1 teaspoon of dried basil

- 1 teaspoon of dried oregano

- Salt and pepper to taste

Directions:

1. Preheat the oven to 375°F (190°C).

2. In a large pot of boiling water, blanch the bell peppers for about 3-4 minutes to soften them slightly. Remove them from the water and set them aside.

3. In a large skillet, heat the olive oil over medium heat. Add the diced onion and minced garlic. Sauté until the onion is translucent and fragrant.

4. Add the diced zucchini and carrot to the skillet and cook for about 5 minutes, or until the vegetables are slightly tender.

5. Stir in the cooked couscous, diced tomatoes (including the juice), dried basil, dried oregano, salt, and pepper. Cook for an additional 2-3 minutes to allow the flavors to combine.

6. Stuff each bell pepper with the couscous and vegetable mixture. Place the stuffed peppers in a baking dish.

7. Sprinkle the grated mozzarella cheese over the stuffed peppers.

8. Cover the baking dish with foil and bake in the preheated oven for 25-30 minutes.

9. Remove the foil and bake for an additional 5-10 minutes, or until the cheese is melted and lightly golden.

10. Garnish the stuffed bell peppers with chopped fresh parsley before serving.

Nutrition:

Stuffed bell peppers with couscous offer a colorful and flavorful dish that combines vegetables, grains, and cheese. Bell peppers are rich in vitamins A and C, while couscous provides carbohydrates and fiber. The addition of vegetables like zucchini and carrots adds nutritional value and texture to the dish. The melted mozzarella cheese adds a creamy and indulgent touch. This recipe is a great way to enjoy a balanced and tasty meal that is both satisfying and nutritious.

CHICKPEA AND SPINACH SALAD:

Preparation time: 10 minutes

Cooking time: 0 minutes

Servings: 4

Ingredients:

- 2 cans (15 ounces each) of chickpeas, drained and rinsed

- 4 cups of fresh spinach leaves

- 1 cup of cherry tomatoes, halved

- 1 cucumber, diced

- 1/2 red onion, thinly sliced

- 1/4 cup of crumbled feta cheese

- Juice of 1 lemon

- 2 tablespoons of olive oil

- 1 teaspoon of dried oregano

- Salt and pepper to taste

Directions:

1. In a large bowl, combine the chickpeas, fresh spinach leaves, halved cherry tomatoes, diced cucumber, thinly sliced red onion, and crumbled feta cheese.

2. In a small bowl, whisk together the lemon juice, olive oil, dried oregano, salt, and pepper to make the dressing.

3. Pour the dressing over the salad ingredients and toss well to combine.

4. Taste and adjust the seasoning if needed.

5. Serve the chickpea and spinach salad immediately as a refreshing and healthy side dish or light lunch.

Nutrition:

Chickpea and spinach salad is a nutritious and satisfying dish that provides a combination of plant-based protein, fiber, and essential vitamins and minerals. Chickpeas are a great source of protein, fiber, and folate, while spinach offers vitamins A and C, iron, and calcium. The addition of fresh vegetables like cherry tomatoes and cucumber adds more vitamins and antioxidants to the salad. The tangy lemon dressing enhances the flavors and adds a refreshing touch. Enjoy this salad as a light and nourishing option.

Roasted Garlic and White Bean Dip:

Preparation time: 10 minutes

Cooking time: 40 minutes

Servings: 6

Ingredients:

- 1 whole garlic bulb

- 2 cans (15 ounces each) of white beans (such as cannellini or great northern), drained and rinsed

- 2 tablespoons of lemon juice

- 2 tablespoons of olive oil

- 1/4 cup of fresh parsley, chopped

- 1/2 teaspoon of dried thyme

- Salt and pepper to taste

Directions:

1. Preheat the oven to 400°F (200°C).

2. Cut off the top of the garlic bulb to expose the cloves. Place the garlic bulb on a piece of aluminum foil and drizzle it with a little olive oil. Wrap the garlic bulb tightly in the foil.

3. Place the wrapped garlic bulb in the preheated oven and roast for about 40 minutes, or until the cloves are soft and golden.

4. Remove the roasted garlic from the oven and allow it to cool slightly. Squeeze the roasted garlic cloves out of their skins and set them aside.

5. In a food processor or blender, combine the roasted garlic cloves, white beans, lemon juice, olive oil, chopped fresh parsley, dried thyme, salt, and pepper.

6. Blend the mixture

GRILLED EGGPLANT ROLL-UPS:

Preparation time: 15 minutes

Cooking time: 10 minutes

Servings: 4

Ingredients:

- 1 large eggplant, sliced lengthwise into thin strips

- 1 cup of ricotta cheese

- 1/4 cup of grated Parmesan cheese

- 2 tablespoons of chopped fresh basil

- 1 clove of garlic, minced

- Salt and pepper to taste

- Olive oil for grilling

Directions:

1. Preheat a grill or grill pan over medium-high heat.

2. Brush the eggplant slices with olive oil on both sides.

3. Grill the eggplant slices for 2-3 minutes per side until they are tender and have grill marks.

4. In a bowl, mix together the ricotta cheese, Parmesan cheese, chopped basil, minced garlic, salt, and pepper.

5. Place a spoonful of the cheese mixture at one end of each grilled eggplant slice and roll it up tightly.

6. Secure each roll-up with a toothpick if necessary.

7. Serve the grilled eggplant roll-ups warm as an appetizer or a side dish.

Quinoa Tabbouleh:

Preparation time: 15 minutes

Cooking time: 15 minutes

Servings: 4

Ingredients:

- 1 cup of cooked quinoa

- 1 cucumber, diced

- 1 tomato, diced

- 1/2 red onion, finely chopped

- 1/4 cup of chopped fresh parsley

- 1/4 cup of chopped fresh mint

- Juice of 1 lemon

- 2 tablespoons of olive oil

- Salt and pepper to taste

Directions:

1. In a large bowl, combine the cooked quinoa, diced cucumber, diced tomato, finely chopped red onion, chopped fresh parsley, and chopped fresh mint.

2. In a separate small bowl, whisk together the lemon juice, olive oil, salt, and pepper to make the dressing.

3. Pour the dressing over the quinoa mixture and toss well to combine.

4. Taste and adjust the seasoning if needed.

5. Let the quinoa tabbouleh sit for a few minutes to allow the flavors to meld.

6. Serve the quinoa tabbouleh chilled as a refreshing and healthy salad.

Baked Zucchini Chips:

Preparation time: 10 minutes

Cooking time: 20 minutes

Servings: 4

Ingredients:

- 2 medium zucchini, sliced into thin rounds

- 1/4 cup of grated Parmesan cheese

- 1/4 cup of breadcrumbs

- 1/2 teaspoon of garlic powder

- 1/2 teaspoon of dried basil

- Salt and pepper to taste

- Olive oil spray

Directions:

1. Preheat the oven to 425°F (220°C). Line a baking sheet with parchment paper.

2. In a shallow bowl, combine the grated Parmesan cheese, breadcrumbs, garlic powder, dried basil, salt, and pepper.

3. Dip each zucchini round into the Parmesan mixture, pressing lightly to coat both sides.

4. Place the coated zucchini rounds on the prepared baking sheet in a single layer.

5. Lightly spray the zucchini rounds with olive oil spray.

6. Bake in the preheated oven for 15-20 minutes, or until the zucchini chips are golden brown and crispy.

7. Remove from the oven and let them cool slightly before serving.

8. Serve the baked zucchini chips as a healthier alternative to traditional potato chips.

EDAMAME AND CORN SALAD:

Preparation time: 10 minutes

Cooking time: 5 minutes

Servings: 4

Ingredients:

- 1 cup of shelled edamame, cooked according to package instructions

- 1 cup of cooked corn kernels

- 1 red bell pepper, diced

- 1/4 cup of chopped red onion

- 1/4 cup of chopped fresh cilantro

- Juice of 1 lime

- 2 tablespoons of olive oil

- 1/2 teaspoon of cumin

- Salt and pepper to taste

Directions:

1. In a large bowl, combine the cooked edamame, cooked corn kernels, diced red bell pepper, chopped red onion, and chopped fresh cilantro.

2. In a separate small bowl, whisk together the lime juice, olive oil, cumin, salt, and pepper to make the dressing.

3. Pour the dressing over the salad ingredients and toss well to combine.

4. Taste and adjust the seasoning if needed.

5. Let the edamame and corn salad sit for a few minutes to allow the flavors to meld.

6. Serve the salad chilled as a nutritious and vibrant side dish.

CARROT GINGER SOUP:

Preparation time: 15 minutes

Cooking time: 25 minutes

Servings: 4

Ingredients:

- 1 tablespoon of olive oil

- 1 onion, diced

- Apologies for the abrupt cutoff. Here's the continuation of the Carrot Ginger Soup recipe:

Ingredients (continued):

- 3 cloves of garlic, minced

- 1 tablespoon of grated fresh ginger

- 4 cups of vegetable broth

- 1 pound of carrots, peeled and chopped

- 1 potato, peeled and chopped

- Salt and pepper to taste

- Optional toppings: fresh cilantro, Greek yogurt, or toasted pumpkin seeds

Directions:

1. In a large pot, heat the olive oil over medium heat.

2. Add the diced onion, minced garlic, and grated ginger to the pot. Sauté for 2-3 minutes until the onion becomes translucent and fragrant.

3. Pour in the vegetable broth and add the chopped carrots and potato.

4. Bring the mixture to a boil and then reduce the heat to low. Cover the pot and simmer for about 20 minutes or until the carrots and potato are tender.

5. Use an immersion blender or transfer the soup to a blender to puree until smooth. Be careful when blending hot liquids.

6. Return the soup to the pot if necessary and season with salt and pepper to taste. Adjust the consistency by adding more broth if desired.

7. Reheat the soup over low heat if needed.

8. Serve the carrot ginger soup hot and garnish with fresh cilantro, a dollop of Greek yogurt, or toasted pumpkin seeds for added flavor and texture.

Enjoy your delicious and healthy meal with these recipes!

Chapter 3

Main Courses

EGGPLANT PARMESAN:

Preparation time: 30 minutes

Cooking time: 45 minutes

Servings: 4

Ingredients:

- 2 large eggplants, sliced into 1/2-inch rounds

- Salt for sprinkling

- 1 cup of all-purpose flour

- 3 eggs, beaten

- 2 cups of breadcrumbs

- 1/2 cup of grated Parmesan cheese

- 2 cups of marinara sauce

- 2 cups of shredded mozzarella cheese

- Fresh basil leaves for garnish

Directions:

1. Preheat the oven to 375°F (190°C). Line a baking sheet with parchment paper.

2. Sprinkle salt on both sides of the eggplant slices and let them sit for about 15 minutes to draw out moisture. Pat the slices dry with a paper towel.

3. Set up three shallow bowls: one with flour, one with beaten eggs, and one with a mixture of breadcrumbs and grated Parmesan cheese.

4. Dredge each eggplant slice in flour, dip it in the beaten eggs, and then coat it with the breadcrumb mixture. Press lightly to adhere the breadcrumbs to the eggplant slice.

5. Place the breaded eggplant slices on the prepared baking sheet in a single layer.

6. Bake the eggplant slices in the preheated oven for 20-25 minutes, or until they are golden brown and crispy.

7. In a baking dish, spread a thin layer of marinara sauce on the bottom. Arrange a layer of baked eggplant slices on top of the sauce.

8. Spoon more marinara sauce over the eggplant slices, followed by a layer of shredded mozzarella cheese. Repeat the layering until all the eggplant slices are used, finishing with a layer of marinara sauce and mozzarella cheese on top.

9. Cover the baking dish with foil and bake in the oven for 20 minutes. Then remove the foil and bake for an additional 10 minutes, or until the cheese is melted and bubbly.

10. Remove from the oven and let it cool for a few minutes before serving. Garnish with fresh basil leaves.

11. Serve the eggplant Parmesan hot as a delicious and satisfying main course.

LENTIL AND VEGETABLE CURRY:

Preparation time: 15 minutes

Cooking time: 30 minutes

Servings: 4

Ingredients:

- 1 cup of dried lentils, rinsed

- 2 tablespoons of vegetable oil

- 1 onion, diced

- 3 cloves of garlic, minced

- 1 tablespoon of grated fresh ginger

- 2 teaspoons of curry powder

- 1 teaspoon of ground cumin

- 1 teaspoon of ground coriander

- 1/2 teaspoon of turmeric

- 1 can (14 ounces) of diced tomatoes

- 1 cup of vegetable broth

- 2 cups of chopped mixed vegetables (such as carrots, bell peppers, zucchini)

- Salt and pepper to taste

- Fresh cilantro for garnish

- Cooked rice or naan bread for serving

Directions:

1. In a saucepan, bring 3 cups of water to a boil. Add the lentils and cook them according to package instructions until tender. Drain and set aside.

2. In a large pot or skillet, heat the vegetable oil over medium heat.

3. Add the diced onion to the pot and sauté for 5 minutes, or until it becomes translucent.

4. Stir in the minced garlic, grated ginger, curry powder, ground cumin, ground coriander, and turmeric. Cook for 1-2 minutes until fragrant.

5. Add the diced tomatoes (with their juice) and vegetable broth to the pot. Stir well to combine.

6. Bring the mixture to a simmer and then add the chopped mixed vegetables and cooked lentils.

7. Season with salt and pepper to taste. Cover the pot and let the curry simmer for about 15 minutes, or until the vegetables are tender.

8. Taste and adjust the seasoning if needed.

9. Garnish the lentil and vegetable curry with fresh cilantro.

10. Serve the curry hot over cooked rice or with naan bread for a satisfying and flavorful meal.

PORTOBELLO MUSHROOM BURGERS:

Preparation time: 15 minutes

Cooking time: 15 minutes

Servings: 4

Ingredients:

- 4 large portobello mushroom caps

- 2 tablespoons of balsamic vinegar

- 2 tablespoons of olive oil

- 2 cloves of garlic, minced

- Salt and pepper to taste

- 4 burger buns

- Toppings of your choice (lettuce, tomato, onion, cheese, etc.)

Directions:

1. Preheat a grill or grill pan over medium-high heat.

2. In a small bowl, whisk together the balsamic vinegar, olive oil, minced garlic, salt, and pepper.

3. Brush both sides of the portobello mushroom caps with the balsamic mixture.

4. Grill the mushroom caps for 4-5 minutes per side, or until they are tender and grill marks appear.

5. While the mushrooms are grilling, toast the burger buns if desired.

6. Place a grilled portobello mushroom cap on each burger bun.

7. Add your choice of toppings, such as lettuce, tomato, onion, and cheese.

8. Serve the portobello mushroom burgers hot and enjoy a delicious vegetarian alternative to traditional burgers.

Quinoa Stuffed Bell Peppers:

Preparation time: 15 minutes

Cooking time: 40 minutes

Servings: 4

Ingredients:

- 4 bell peppers (any color), tops removed and seeds removed

- 1 cup of cooked quinoa

- 1/2 cup of black beans, rinsed and drained

- 1/2 cup of corn kernels

- 1/2 cup of diced tomatoes

- 1/4 cup of chopped fresh cilantro

- 1/4 cup of shredded cheddar cheese

- 1 teaspoon of chili powder

- 1/2 teaspoon of cumin

- Salt and pepper to taste

Directions:

1. Preheat the oven to 375°F (190°C). Grease a baking dish that can hold the bell peppers upright.

2. In a large bowl, combine the cooked quinoa, black beans, corn kernels, diced tomatoes, chopped cilantro, shredded cheddar cheese, chili powder, cumin, salt, and pepper. Mix well to combine.

3. Stuff each bell pepper with the quinoa mixture, pressing it down gently.

4. Place the stuffed bell peppers in the prepared baking dish.

5. Bake in the preheated oven for 30-35 minutes, or until the bell peppers are tender and the filling is heated through.

6. Remove from the oven and let them cool for a few minutes before serving.

7. Serve the quinoa stuffed bell peppers as a nutritious and flavorful main course.

Sweet Potato and Chickpea Stew:

Preparation time: 15 minutes

Cooking time: 30 minutes

Servings: 4

Ingredients:

- 2 tablespoons of olive oil

- 1 onion, diced

- 3 cloves of garlic, minced

- 1 tablespoon of grated fresh ginger

- 2 teaspoons of ground cumin

- 1 teaspoon of ground coriander

- 1/2 teaspoon of turmeric

- 1/4 teaspoon of cinnamon

- 2 medium sweet potatoes, peeled and diced

- 1 can (14 ounces) of diced tomatoes

- 1 can (14 ounces) of chickpeas, rinsed and drained

- 2 cups of vegetable broth

- Salt and pepper to taste

- Fresh cilantro for garnish

Directions:

1. In a large pot, heat the olive oil over medium heat.

2. Add the diced onion to the pot and sauté for 5 minutes, or until it becomes translucent.

3. Stir in the minced garlic, grated ginger, ground cumin, ground coriander, turmeric, and cinnamon. Cook for 1-2 minutes until fragrant.

4. Add the diced sweet potatoes, diced tomatoes (with their juice), chickpeas, and vegetable broth to the pot. Stir well to combine.

5. Bring the mixture to a boil and then reduce the heat to low. Cover the pot and simmer for about 20-25 minutes, or until the sweet potatoes are tender.

6. Season with salt and pepper to taste.

7. Garnish the sweet potato and chickpea stew with fresh cilantro.

8. Serve the stew hot and enjoy a hearty and comforting meal.

Enjoy these delicious and satisfying vegetarian recipes

Spinach and Ricotta Stuffed Shells:

Preparation time: 30 minutes

Cooking time: 35 minutes

Servings: 4-6

Ingredients:

- 20 jumbo pasta shells

- 2 cups of ricotta cheese

- 1 cup of shredded mozzarella cheese, divided

- 1/2 cup of grated Parmesan cheese

- 1 large egg

- 2 cups of fresh spinach, chopped

- 2 cloves of garlic, minced

- 1 teaspoon of dried basil

- 1 teaspoon of dried oregano

- Salt and pepper to taste

- 2 cups of marinara sauce

Directions:

1. Preheat the oven to 375°F (190°C). Grease a baking dish that can hold the stuffed shells in a single layer.

2. Cook the jumbo pasta shells according to the package instructions until al dente. Drain and set aside.

3. In a large bowl, combine the ricotta cheese, 1/2 cup of shredded mozzarella cheese, grated Parmesan cheese, egg, chopped spinach, minced garlic, dried basil, dried oregano, salt, and pepper. Mix well.

4. Spoon the spinach and ricotta mixture into each cooked pasta shell and place them in the prepared baking dish.

5. Pour the marinara sauce over the stuffed shells, ensuring that they are well covered.

6. Cover the baking dish with foil and bake in the preheated oven for 20 minutes.

7. Remove the foil, sprinkle the remaining 1/2 cup of shredded mozzarella cheese over the shells, and bake for an additional 15 minutes, or until the cheese is melted and bubbly.

8. Remove from the oven and let it cool for a few minutes before serving.

9. Serve the spinach and ricotta stuffed shells hot as a delicious and comforting meal.

TOFU STIR-FRY WITH VEGETABLES:

Preparation time: 15 minutes

Cooking time: 15 minutes

Servings: 4

Ingredients:

- 14 ounces of firm tofu, drained and cubed

- 2 tablespoons of soy sauce

- 1 tablespoon of hoisin sauce

- 1 tablespoon of rice vinegar

- 1 tablespoon of cornstarch

- 1 tablespoon of vegetable oil

- 1 onion, thinly sliced

- 2 bell peppers, thinly sliced

- 2 cups of broccoli florets

- 1 cup of sliced mushrooms

- 2 cloves of garlic, minced

- 1 tablespoon of grated fresh ginger

- Salt and pepper to taste

- Cooked rice or noodles for serving

Directions:

1. In a small bowl, whisk together the soy sauce, hoisin sauce, rice vinegar, and cornstarch to make a sauce. Set aside.

2. Heat the vegetable oil in a large skillet or wok over medium-high heat.

3. Add the cubed tofu to the skillet and cook until it becomes golden brown and crispy on all sides. Remove the tofu from the skillet and set aside.

4. In the same skillet, add the sliced onion, bell peppers, broccoli florets, and sliced mushrooms. Stir-fry for 3-4 minutes, or until the vegetables are crisp-tender.

5. Add the minced garlic and grated ginger to the skillet and stir-fry for an additional minute.

6. Return the tofu to the skillet and pour the sauce over the tofu and vegetables. Stir well to coat everything evenly.

7. Cook for another 2-3 minutes, or until the sauce thickens and coats the tofu and vegetables.

8. Season with salt and pepper to taste.

9. Serve the tofu stir-fry hot over cooked rice or noodles for a flavorful and nutritious meal.

RATATOUILLE:

Preparation time: 20 minutes

Cooking time: 40 minutes

Servings: 4-6

Ingredients:

- 2 tablespoons of olive oil

- 1 onion, diced

- 3 cloves of garlic, minced

- 1 eggplant, diced

- 2 zucchini, diced

- 1 red bell pepper, diced

- 1 yellow bell pepper, diced

- 1 can (14 ounces) of diced tomatoes

- 2 tablespoons of tomato paste

- 1 teaspoon of dried thyme

- 1 teaspoon of dried oregano

- Salt and pepper to taste

- Fresh basil leaves for garnish

Directions:

1. Heat the olive oil in a large pot or skillet over medium heat.

2. Add the diced onion to the pot and sauté for 5 minutes, or until it becomes translucent.

3. Stir in the minced garlic and cook for an additional minute.

4. Add the diced eggplant, diced zucchini, diced red bell pepper, and diced yellow bell pepper to the pot. Stir well to combine.

5. Cook the vegetables for about 10 minutes, or until they start to soften.

6. Add the diced tomatoes and tomato paste to the pot. Stir well to combine.

7. Season with dried thyme, dried oregano, salt, and pepper. Stir again.

8. Reduce the heat to low, cover the pot, and simmer for 20-25 minutes, or until the vegetables are tender and the flavors have melded together.

9. Taste and adjust the seasoning if needed.

10. Serve the ratatouille hot, garnished with fresh basil leaves. It can be enjoyed as a side dish or served over cooked rice, pasta, or crusty bread.

SPINACH AND MUSHROOM LASAGNA:

Preparation time: 30 minutes

Cooking time: 1 hour

Servings: 6-8

Ingredients:

- 12 lasagna noodles

- 2 tablespoons of olive oil

- 1 onion, diced

- 3 cloves of garlic, minced

- 8 ounces of mushrooms, sliced

- 4 cups of fresh spinach

- 2 cups of ricotta cheese

- 1/2 cup of grated Parmesan cheese

- 2 cups of shredded mozzarella cheese, divided

- 2 cups of marinara sauce

- 1 teaspoon of dried basil

- 1 teaspoon of dried oregano

- Salt and pepper to taste

Directions:

1. Preheat the oven to 375°F (190°C). Grease a 9x13-inch baking dish.

2. Cook the lasagna noodles according to the package instructions until al dente. Drain and set aside.

3. In a large skillet, heat the olive oil over medium heat.

4. Add the diced onion and minced garlic to the skillet and sauté for 5 minutes, or until the onion becomes translucent.

5. Add the sliced mushrooms to the skillet and cook for another 5 minutes, or until they release their moisture and start to brown.

6. Add the fresh spinach to the skillet and cook until it wilts.

7. In a separate bowl, combine the ricotta cheese, grated Parmesan cheese, 1 cup of shredded mozzarella cheese, dried basil, dried oregano, salt, and pepper. Mix well.

8. Spread a thin layer of marinara sauce on the bottom of the prepared baking dish.

9. Arrange 4 lasagna noodles over the sauce, slightly overlapping them.

10. Spread half of the spinach and mushroom mixture over the noodles, followed by half of the ricotta cheese mixture.

11. Repeat the layers with 4 more lasagna noodles, the remaining spinach and mushroom mixture, and the remaining ricotta cheese mixture.

12. Top with the remaining 4 lasagna noodles and pour the remaining marinara sauce over them.

13. Sprinkle the remaining 1 cup of shredded mozzarella cheese over the lasagna.

14. Cover the baking dish with foil and bake in the preheated oven for 30 minutes.

15. Remove the foil and bake for an additional 15 minutes, or until the cheese is melted and golden brown.

16. Remove from the oven and let it cool for a few minutes before serving.

17. Serve the spinach and mushroom lasagna hot as a hearty and flavorful meal.

BLACK BEAN AND QUINOA ENCHILADAS:

Preparation time: 30 minutes

Cooking time: 25 minutes

Servings: 4-6

Ingredients:

- 1 cup of cooked quinoa

- 1 can (15 ounces) of black beans, rinsed and drained

- 1 cup of corn kernels (fresh or frozen)

- 1/2 cup of diced red bell pepper

- 1/2 cup of diced green bell pepper

- 1/2 cup of diced onion

- 2 cloves of garlic, minced

- 1 tablespoon of olive oil

- 1 teaspoon of ground cumin

- 1 teaspoon of chili powder

- Salt and pepper to taste

- 2 cups of enchilada sauce

- 8-10 corn tortillas

- 1 cup of shredded cheddar cheese

- Fresh cilantro leaves for garnish (optional)

Directions:

1. Preheat the oven to 375°F (190°C). Grease a baking dish that can hold the enchiladas in a single layer.

2. In a large bowl, combine the cooked quinoa, black beans, corn kernels, diced red bell pepper, diced green bell pepper, diced onion, minced garlic, olive oil, ground cumin, chili powder, salt, and pepper. Mix well.

3. Pour 1/2 cup of enchilada sauce into the bottom of the prepared baking dish.

4. Warm the corn tortillas in the microwave or on a hot skillet to make them pliable.

5. Spoon a generous amount of the quinoa and black bean mixture onto each tortilla and roll it up. Place the rolled enchiladas in the baking dish, seam side down.

6. Pour the remaining enchilada sauce over the

FALAFEL WITH TAHINI SAUCE:

Preparation time: 20 minutes

Cooking time: 15 minutes

Servings: 4-6

Ingredients:

For the falafel:

- 2 cups of cooked chickpeas

- 1/2 cup of fresh parsley leaves

- 1/2 cup of fresh cilantro leaves

- 3 cloves of garlic

- 1 small onion, roughly chopped

- 2 tablespoons of all-purpose flour

- 1 teaspoon of ground cumin

- 1 teaspoon of ground coriander

- 1/2 teaspoon of baking powder

- Salt and pepper to taste

- Vegetable oil for frying

For the tahini sauce:

- 1/2 cup of tahini paste

- 2 tablespoons of fresh lemon juice

- 2 tablespoons of water

- 1 clove of garlic, minced

- Salt to taste

For serving:

- Pita bread or wraps

- Lettuce, tomatoes, cucumbers, and any other desired toppings

Directions:

1. In a food processor, combine the cooked chickpeas, parsley, cilantro, garlic, onion, flour, cumin, coriander, baking powder, salt, and pepper. Pulse until well combined and the mixture comes together, but still has some texture.

2. Shape the falafel mixture into small patties or balls, about the size of a golf ball.

3. Heat vegetable oil in a frying pan over medium heat. Fry the falafel in batches until golden brown and crispy on all sides. Remove from the pan and drain on a paper towel-lined plate.

4. In a small bowl, whisk together the tahini paste, lemon juice, water, minced garlic, and salt until smooth and creamy. Add more water if needed to achieve the desired consistency.

5. Serve the falafel in pita bread or wraps, topped with lettuce, tomatoes, cucumbers, and any other desired toppings. Drizzle with the tahini sauce and enjoy!

BUTTERNUT SQUASH RISOTTO:

Preparation time: 10 minutes

Cooking time: 40 minutes

Servings: 4

Ingredients:

- 1 butternut squash, peeled, seeded, and diced

- 4 cups of vegetable broth

- 2 tablespoons of olive oil

- 1 onion, finely chopped

- 2 cloves of garlic, minced

- 1 1/2 cups of Arborio rice

- 1/2 cup of white wine (optional)

- 1/2 teaspoon of dried thyme

- Salt and pepper to taste

- 1/2 cup of grated Parmesan cheese

- Fresh parsley leaves for garnish

Directions:

1. In a large pot, bring the vegetable broth to a simmer. Keep it warm over low heat.

2. In a separate large pot or deep skillet, heat the olive oil over medium heat.

3. Add the chopped onion and minced garlic to the pot and sauté for 5 minutes, or until the onion becomes translucent.

4. Add the diced butternut squash to the pot and cook for another 5 minutes, stirring occasionally.

5. Stir in the Arborio rice and cook for 1-2 minutes, until the rice is well coated with the oil and starts to become translucent around the edges.

6. If using, pour in the white wine and cook until it is absorbed by the rice.

7. Begin adding the warm vegetable broth to the pot, one ladleful at a time, stirring continuously and allowing each ladleful to be absorbed before adding the next.

8. Continue adding broth and stirring until the rice is tender and creamy but still slightly firm to the bite (al dente). This process will take about 20-25 minutes.

9. Stir in the dried thyme, salt, and pepper.

10. Remove the pot from the heat and stir in the grated Parmesan cheese until it melts and combines with the risotto.

11. Let the risotto rest for a few minutes to allow it to thicken.

12. Serve the butternut squash risotto hot, garnished with fresh parsley leaves.

VEGGIE PAD THAI:

Preparation time: 20 minutes

Cooking time: 15 minutes

Servings: 4

Ingredients:

- 8 ounces of rice noodles

- 2 tablespoons of vegetable oil

- 1 onion, thinly sliced

- 2 cloves of garlic, minced

- 1 red bell pepper, thinly sliced

- 1 carrot, julienned or thinly sliced

- 1 zucchini, julienned or thinly sliced

- 1 cup of bean sprouts

- 2 green onions, chopped

- 1/4 cup of chopped peanuts

- Fresh cilantro leaves for garnish (optional)

- Lime wedges for serving

For the sauce:

- 3 tablespoons of soy sauce

- 2 tablespoons of tamarind paste

- 2 tablespoons of lime juice

- 2 tablespoons of brown sugar

- 1 tablespoon of rice vinegar

- 1 tablespoon of Sriracha sauce (optional)

Directions:

1. Cook the rice noodles according to the package instructions. Drain and set aside.

2. In a small bowl, whisk together the soy sauce, tamarind paste, lime juice, brown sugar, rice vinegar, and Sriracha sauce to make the sauce. Set aside.

3. Heat the vegetable oil in a large skillet or wok over medium-high heat.

4. Add the sliced onion and minced garlic to the skillet and sauté for 2-3 minutes until the onion becomes translucent.

5. Add the sliced bell pepper, julienned carrot, and zucchini to the skillet. Stir-fry for another 3-4 minutes until the vegetables are crisp-tender.

6. Push the vegetables to one side of the skillet and crack the eggs into the empty space. Scramble the eggs with a spatula until cooked through.

7. Add the cooked rice noodles to the skillet along with the bean sprouts and chopped green onions. Pour the sauce over the noodles and vegetables.

8. Toss everything together until well combined and heated through.

9. Remove from heat and garnish with chopped peanuts and fresh cilantro leaves, if desired.

10. Serve the veggie pad Thai hot, with lime wedges on the side for squeezing over the dish.

MUSHROOM AND SPINACH QUESADILLAS:

Preparation time: 10 minutes

Cooking time: 15 minutes

Servings: 4

Ingredients:

- 8 small flour tortillas

- 2 cups of sliced mushrooms

- 2 cups of fresh spinach leaves

- 1 small onion, thinly sliced

- 2 cloves of garlic, minced

- 1 cup of shredded cheese (such as mozzarella, cheddar, or Monterey Jack)

- 2 tablespoons of olive oil

- Salt and pepper to taste

- Salsa, guacamole, or sour cream for serving (optional)

Directions:

1. Heat one tablespoon of olive oil in a large skillet over medium-high heat.

2. Add the sliced mushrooms to the skillet and cook for 5-6 minutes until they release their moisture and start to brown. Remove from the skillet and set aside.

3. In the same skillet, add the remaining tablespoon of olive oil and sauté the sliced onion and minced garlic until the onion becomes translucent, about 3-4 minutes.

4. Add the fresh spinach leaves to the skillet and cook until wilted, about 2-3 minutes. Season with salt and pepper.

5. Remove the spinach mixture from the skillet and set aside.

6. Place a tortilla on a clean surface and sprinkle a small amount of shredded cheese on one half of the tortilla.

7. Top the cheese with a portion of the cooked mushrooms and spinach mixture.

8. Fold the tortilla in half to cover the filling.

9. Repeat steps 6-8 with the remaining tortillas and filling ingredients.

10. Heat a clean skillet or griddle over medium heat. Cook each quesadilla for 2-3 minutes on each side until the cheese is melted and the tortilla is golden brown.

11. Remove from heat and cut each quesadilla into wedges.

12. Serve the mushroom and spinach quesadillas hot, with salsa, guacamole, or sour cream on the side for dipping, if desired.

Lentil Shepherd's Pie:

Preparation time: 20 minutes

Cooking time: 45 minutes

Servings: 6

Ingredients:

For the lentil filling:

- 1 cup of dried green lentils

- 3 cups of vegetable broth

- 1 tablespoon of olive oil

- 1 onion, diced

- 2 cloves of garlic, minced

- 2 carrots, diced

- 2 celery stalks, diced

- 1 cup of frozen peas

- 1 teaspoon of dried thyme

- 1 teaspoon of dried rosemary

- Salt and pepper to taste

For the mashed potato topping:

- 4 large potatoes, peeled and cut into chunks

- 1/2 cup of unsweetened plant-based milk (such as almond or soy milk)

- 2 tablespoons of vegan butter

- Salt and pepper to taste

Directions:

1. Rinse the lentils under cold water and drain.

2. In a large pot, combine the lentils and vegetable broth. Bring to a boil, then reduce the heat and simmer for about 20-25 minutes, or until the lentils are tender. Drain any excess liquid and set aside.

3. In the same pot, heat the olive oil over medium heat. Add the diced onion and minced garlic and sauté for 5 minutes, until the onion becomes translucent.

4. Add the diced carrots and celery to the pot and cook for another 5 minutes

Chapter 4

Pasta & Grains

Zucchini Noodles with Avocado Pesto:

Preparation time: 15 minutes

Cooking time: 0 minutes

Servings: 2

Ingredients:

- 2 medium-sized zucchini

- 1 ripe avocado

- 1/2 cup fresh basil leaves

- 2 cloves of garlic

- 2 tablespoons of pine nuts

- 2 tablespoons of lemon juice

- 2 tablespoons of olive oil

- Salt and pepper to taste

- Optional toppings: cherry tomatoes, grated Parmesan cheese, additional pine nuts

Directions:

1. Using a spiralizer or a vegetable peeler, cut the zucchini into thin noodle-like strips.

2. Place the zucchini noodles in a large bowl.

3. In a food processor or blender, combine the avocado, basil leaves, garlic, pine nuts, lemon juice, olive oil, salt, and pepper. Blend until smooth and creamy.

4. Pour the avocado pesto over the zucchini noodles and toss until the noodles are well coated.

5. Serve the zucchini noodles with avocado pesto as is or top with cherry tomatoes, grated Parmesan cheese, and additional pine nuts if desired.

STUFFED ACORN SQUASH:

Preparation time: 20 minutes

Cooking time: 50 minutes

Servings: 4

Ingredients:

- 2 acorn squash

- 1 tablespoon of olive oil

- 1 onion, diced

- 2 cloves of garlic, minced

- 1 red bell pepper, diced

- 1 zucchini, diced

- 1 cup of cooked quinoa

- 1/2 cup of dried cranberries

- 1/2 cup of chopped walnuts

- 1 teaspoon of dried thyme

- Salt and pepper to taste

Directions:

1. Preheat the oven to 375°F (190°C).

2. Cut the acorn squash in half lengthwise and scoop out the seeds and membranes.

3. Place the squash halves cut side down on a baking sheet and bake for 30 minutes, or until the squash is tender when pierced with a fork.

4. While the squash is baking, heat the olive oil in a large skillet over medium heat.

5. Add the diced onion and minced garlic to the skillet and sauté for 5 minutes until the onion becomes translucent.

6. Add the diced red bell pepper and zucchini to the skillet and cook for another 5 minutes until the vegetables are tender.

7. Stir in the cooked quinoa, dried cranberries, chopped walnuts, dried thyme, salt, and pepper. Cook for 2-3 minutes to allow the flavors to blend.

8. Remove the squash halves from the oven and flip them over. Fill each squash half with the quinoa and vegetable mixture, packing it tightly.

9. Return the stuffed squash halves to the oven and bake for an additional 15-20 minutes, until the filling is heated through and the tops are slightly browned.

10. Serve the stuffed acorn squash as a main dish or as a side dish.

Spinach and Feta Stuffed Portobello Mushrooms:

Preparation time: 15 minutes

Cooking time: 20 minutes

Servings: 4

Ingredients:

- 4 large Portobello mushrooms

- 2 tablespoons of olive oil

- 2 cloves of garlic, minced

- 4 cups of fresh spinach leaves

- 1/2 cup of crumbled feta cheese

- Salt and pepper to taste

Directions:

1. Preheat the oven to 375°F (190°C).

2. Remove the stems and gills from the Portobello mushrooms and wipe them clean with a damp cloth.

3. Place the mushrooms on a baking sheet, gill-side up.

4. In a large skillet, heat the olive oil over medium heat.

5. Add the minced garlic to the skillet and sauté for 1 minute until fragrant.

6. Add the fresh spinach leaves to the skillet and cook until wilted, about 2-3 minutes. Season with salt and pepper.

7. Divide the sautéed spinach evenly among the Portobello mushrooms, filling the gill-side cavity.

8. Sprinkle the crumbled feta cheese over the spinach in each mushroom.

9. Bake the stuffed Portobello mushrooms in the preheated oven for 15-20 minutes, until the mushrooms are tender and the cheese is slightly browned.

10. Serve the spinach and feta stuffed Portobello mushrooms as a main dish or as a side dish.

Sweet Potato and Black Bean Burritos:

Preparation time: 20 minutes

Cooking time: 30 minutes

Servings: 4

Ingredients:

- 2 medium-sized sweet potatoes, peeled and diced

- 1 tablespoon of olive oil

- 1 onion, diced

- 2 cloves of garlic, minced

- 1 teaspoon of ground cumin

- 1/2 teaspoon of chili powder- 1/2 teaspoon of paprika

- 1 can (15 ounces) of black beans, rinsed and drained

- Salt and pepper to taste

- 4 large flour tortillas

- Optional toppings: salsa, avocado slices, sour cream, shredded cheese, cilantro

Directions:

1. Place the diced sweet potatoes in a microwave-safe bowl and microwave on high for 5-7 minutes, or until the sweet potatoes are tender.

2. In a large skillet, heat the olive oil over medium heat.

3. Add the diced onion and minced garlic to the skillet and sauté for 5 minutes until the onion becomes translucent.

4. Add the cooked sweet potatoes, ground cumin, chili powder, and paprika to the skillet. Stir to coat the sweet potatoes with the spices.

5. Add the black beans to the skillet and season with salt and pepper. Cook for an additional 2-3 minutes to heat the beans through.

6. Warm the flour tortillas in a dry skillet or in the microwave.

7. Place a scoop of the sweet potato and black bean mixture onto each tortilla, slightly off-center.

8. Add desired toppings such as salsa, avocado slices, sour cream, shredded cheese, and cilantro.

9. Fold the sides of the tortilla over the filling, then roll it up tightly.

10. Serve the sweet potato and black bean burritos as is or lightly grill them in a skillet to crisp up the tortilla.

Quinoa and Vegetable Stir-Fry:

Preparation time: 15 minutes

Cooking time: 20 minutes

Servings: 4

Ingredients:

- 1 cup of quinoa

- 2 cups of vegetable broth or water

- 2 tablespoons of olive oil

- 1 onion, diced

- 2 cloves of garlic, minced

- 1 red bell pepper, diced

- 1 zucchini, diced

- 1 cup of broccoli florets

- 1 cup of snap peas

- 1 carrot, julienned

- 3 tablespoons of soy sauce or tamari

- 2 tablespoons of rice vinegar

- 1 tablespoon of honey or maple syrup

- 1 teaspoon of sesame oil

- Optional toppings: chopped green onions, sesame seeds

Directions:

1. Rinse the quinoa under cold water in a fine-mesh sieve.

2. In a medium saucepan, bring the vegetable broth or water to a boil. Add the rinsed quinoa, reduce the heat to low, cover, and simmer for 15 minutes, or until the quinoa is cooked and the liquid is absorbed. Remove from heat and let it sit covered for 5 minutes. Fluff the quinoa with a fork.

3. In a large skillet or wok, heat the olive oil over medium heat.

4. Add the diced onion and minced garlic to the skillet and sauté for 5 minutes until the onion becomes translucent.

5. Add the diced red bell pepper, zucchini, broccoli florets, snap peas, and julienned carrot to the skillet. Stir-fry for 5-7 minutes until the vegetables are tender-crisp.

6. In a small bowl, whisk together the soy sauce or tamari, rice vinegar, honey or maple syrup, and sesame oil.

7. Pour the sauce over the stir-fried vegetables and toss to coat evenly.

8. Add the cooked quinoa to the skillet and stir-fry for an additional 2-3 minutes until the quinoa is heated through.

9. Remove from heat and garnish with chopped green onions and sesame seeds if desired.

10. Serve the quinoa and vegetable stir-fry as a main dish or as a side dish.

Enjoy your delicious and healthy meals

Spaghetti Aglio e Olio:

Preparation time: 10 minutes

Cooking time: 15 minutes

Servings: 4

Ingredients:

- 12 ounces (340g) of spaghetti

- 1/3 cup of olive oil

- 6 cloves of garlic, thinly sliced

- 1/2 teaspoon of red pepper flakes (adjust to taste)

- Salt to taste

- 1/4 cup of chopped fresh parsley

- Grated Parmesan cheese for serving (optional)

Directions:

1. Cook the spaghetti according to the package instructions until al dente. Drain and set aside.

2. In a large skillet, heat the olive oil over medium heat.

3. Add the sliced garlic and red pepper flakes to the skillet. Cook for 2-3 minutes, stirring occasionally, until the garlic is lightly golden and fragrant. Be careful not to burn the garlic.

4. Add the cooked spaghetti to the skillet and toss well to coat the pasta with the garlic-infused oil.

5. Season with salt to taste and sprinkle the chopped parsley over the spaghetti. Toss again to combine.

6. Remove from heat and serve the spaghetti aglio e olio immediately, with grated Parmesan cheese on top if desired.

MUSHROOM RISOTTO:

Preparation time: 10 minutes

Cooking time: 30 minutes

Servings: 4

Ingredients:

- 1 tablespoon of olive oil

- 1 onion, finely chopped

- 2 cloves of garlic, minced

- 8 ounces (225g) of mushrooms, sliced

- 1 cup of Arborio rice

- 1/2 cup of white wine (optional)

- 4 cups of vegetable broth, heated

- 1/2 cup of grated Parmesan cheese

- 2 tablespoons of butter

- Salt and pepper to taste

- Chopped fresh parsley for garnish (optional)

Directions:

1. In a large saucepan, heat the olive oil over medium heat.

2. Add the chopped onion and minced garlic to the saucepan. Sauté for 2-3 minutes until the onion becomes translucent.

3. Add the sliced mushrooms to the saucepan and cook for another 5 minutes until the mushrooms are tender and slightly browned.

4. Add the Arborio rice to the saucepan and stir to coat the rice with the oil and mushrooms. Cook for 1-2 minutes until the rice grains are translucent around the edges.

5. If using, pour in the white wine and stir until it is absorbed by the rice.

6. Add a ladleful of heated vegetable broth to the saucepan and stir until the liquid is absorbed by the rice. Continue adding the broth, one ladleful at a time, stirring constantly and allowing the rice to absorb the liquid before adding more. Cook until the rice is creamy and al dente, about 20-25 minutes.

7. Stir in the grated Parmesan cheese and butter until melted and well combined. Season with salt and pepper to taste.

8. Remove from heat and let the risotto rest for a few minutes.

9. Serve the mushroom risotto hot, garnished with chopped fresh parsley if desired.

Pesto Pasta with Cherry Tomatoes:

Preparation time: 10 minutes

Cooking time: 10 minutes

Servings: 4

Ingredients:

- 12 ounces (340g) of pasta (such as fusilli or penne)

- 1 cup of fresh basil leaves

- 1/4 cup of pine nuts

- 2 cloves of garlic

- 1/2 cup of grated Parmesan cheese

- 1/3 cup of olive oil

- Salt and pepper to taste

- 1 cup of cherry tomatoes, halved

Directions:

1. Cook the pasta according to the package instructions until al dente. Drain and set aside.

2. In a food processor or blender, combine the fresh basil leaves, pine nuts, garlic, grated Parmesan cheese, olive oil, salt, and pepper. Blend until smooth and creamy.

3. In a large skillet, heat a drizzle of olive oil over medium heat.

4. Add the halved cherry tomatoes to the skillet and cook for 2-3 minutes until they start to soften.

5. Add the cooked pasta to the skillet and pour the pesto sauce over the pasta. Toss well to coat the pasta with the sauce and warm it up.

6. Remove from heat and serve the pesto pasta with cherry tomatoes immediately.

VEGETABLE FRIED RICE:

Preparation time: 10 minutes

Cooking time: 15 minutes

Servings: 4

Ingredients:

- 3 cups of cooked rice (preferably cooled or day-old rice)

- 2 tablespoons of vegetable oil

- 1 onion, diced

- 2 cloves of garlic, minced

- 1 carrot, diced

- 1 cup of frozen peas

- 1 red bell pepper, diced

- 2 eggs- Pesto Pasta with Cherry Tomatoes (continued):

7. Heat the vegetable oil in a large skillet or wok over medium heat.

8. Add the diced onion and minced garlic to the skillet and sauté for 2-3 minutes until the onion becomes translucent.

9. Add the diced carrot, frozen peas, and diced red bell pepper to the skillet. Cook for another 3-4 minutes until the vegetables are tender-crisp.

10. Push the vegetables to one side of the skillet and crack the eggs into the empty space. Scramble the eggs with a spatula until they are cooked through.

11. Mix the scrambled eggs with the vegetables in the skillet.

12. Add the cooked rice to the skillet and stir-fry everything together for 2-3 minutes until the rice is heated through and well combined with the vegetables and eggs.

13. Pour the soy sauce and sesame oil over the fried rice and stir-fry for another minute.

14. Remove from heat and serve the vegetable fried rice hot.

Caprese Pasta Salad:

Preparation time: 15 minutes

Cooking time: 10 minutes (for pasta)

Servings: 4

Ingredients:

- 8 ounces (225g) of pasta (such as penne or fusilli)

- 1 cup of cherry tomatoes, halved

- 8 ounces (225g) of fresh mozzarella cheese, cubed

- 1/2 cup of fresh basil leaves, torn

- 2 tablespoons of extra virgin olive oil

- 2 tablespoons of balsamic vinegar

- Salt and pepper to taste

Directions:

1. Cook the pasta according to the package instructions until al dente. Drain and rinse with cold water to cool the pasta down.

2. In a large bowl, combine the cooked pasta, cherry tomatoes, fresh mozzarella cheese, and torn basil leaves.

3. Drizzle the extra virgin olive oil and balsamic vinegar over the pasta salad. Season with salt and pepper to taste.

4. Toss everything together until well combined and evenly coated with the dressing.

5. Let the Caprese pasta salad sit for a few minutes to allow the flavors to meld.

6. Serve the salad at room temperature or chilled.

Enjoy your meal

SPINACH AND RICOTTA STUFFED SHELLS:

Preparation time: 15 minutes

Cooking time: 30 minutes

Servings: 4

Ingredients:

- 20 jumbo pasta shells

- 2 cups of ricotta cheese

- 1 cup of frozen spinach, thawed and squeezed dry

- 1 cup of shredded mozzarella cheese

- 1/2 cup of grated Parmesan cheese

- 1 egg

- 2 cloves of garlic, minced

- 1 teaspoon of dried basil

- 1 teaspoon of dried oregano

- Salt and pepper to taste

- 2 cups of marinara sauce

Directions:

1. Preheat the oven to 350°F (175°C).

2. Cook the jumbo pasta shells according to the package instructions until al dente. Drain and set aside.

3. In a mixing bowl, combine the ricotta cheese, thawed spinach, shredded mozzarella cheese, grated Parmesan cheese, egg, minced garlic, dried basil, dried oregano, salt, and pepper. Mix well until all ingredients are evenly incorporated.

4. Spread a thin layer of marinara sauce on the bottom of a baking dish.

5. Stuff each cooked pasta shell with the spinach and ricotta mixture and place them in the baking dish.

6. Pour the remaining marinara sauce over the stuffed shells, covering them completely.

7. Cover the baking dish with foil and bake in the preheated oven for 20 minutes.

8. Remove the foil and continue baking for an additional 10 minutes until the cheese on top is melted and bubbly.

9. Let the stuffed shells cool for a few minutes before serving.

Quinoa Tabbouleh Salad:

Preparation time: 15 minutes

Cooking time: 15 minutes (for quinoa)

Servings: 4

Ingredients:

- 1 cup of quinoa

- 2 cups of water

- 1 cup of chopped fresh parsley

- 1/2 cup of chopped fresh mint leaves

- 1 cucumber, seeded and diced

- 2 tomatoes, diced

- 1/4 cup of finely chopped red onion

- Juice of 1 lemon

- 3 tablespoons of extra virgin olive oil

- Salt and pepper to taste

Directions:

1. Rinse the quinoa thoroughly under cold water.

2. In a saucepan, bring the water to a boil. Add the rinsed quinoa and reduce the heat to low. Cover and simmer for about 15 minutes until the quinoa is cooked and the water is absorbed.

3. Fluff the cooked quinoa with a fork and let it cool.

4. In a large bowl, combine the chopped parsley, chopped mint leaves, diced cucumber, diced tomatoes, and finely chopped red onion.

5. Add the cooked and cooled quinoa to the bowl and mix well.

6. In a small separate bowl, whisk together the lemon juice, extra virgin olive oil, salt, and pepper.

7. Pour the dressing over the quinoa tabbouleh salad and toss to coat all the ingredients.

8. Adjust the seasoning if needed.

9. Let the salad sit for a few minutes before serving to allow the flavors to meld.

Lemon Garlic Orzo:

Preparation time: 5 minutes

Cooking time: 15 minutes

Servings: 4

Ingredients:

- 1 cup of orzo pasta

- 2 tablespoons of butter

- 2 cloves of garlic, minced

- Zest of 1 lemon

- Juice of 1 lemon

- 1/4 cup of grated Parmesan cheese

- Salt and pepper to taste

- Chopped fresh parsley for garnish (optional)

Directions:

1. Cook the orzo pasta according to the package instructions until al dente. Drain and set aside.

2. In a large skillet, melt the butter over medium heat.

3. Add the minced garlic to the skillet and sauté for 1-2 minutes until fragrant.

4. Add the cooked orzo to the skillet and toss to coat the pasta with the garlic-infused butter.

5. Add the lemon zest and lemon juice to the skillet and stir to combine.

6. Stir in the grated Parmesan cheese until melted and well distributed.

7. Season with salt and pepper to taste.

8. Remove from heat and garnish with chopped fresh parsley if desired.

9. Serve the lemon garlic orzo hot.

ROASTED VEGETABLE COUSCOUS:

Preparation time: 15 minutes

Cooking time: 25 minutes

Servings: 4

Ingredients:

- 1 cup of couscous

- 1 1/2 cups of vegetable broth

- 1 red bell pepper, diced

- 1 zucchini, diced

- 1 yellow squash, diced

- 1 red onion, sliced

- 2 tablespoons of olive oil

- 1 teaspoon of dried thyme

- 1 teaspoon of dried oregano

- Salt and pepper to taste

- Fresh parsley for garnish (optional)

Directions:

1. Preheat the oven to 400°F (200°C).

2. In a large baking sheet, toss the diced red bell pepper, zucchini, yellow squash, and sliced red onion with olive oil, dried thyme, dried oregano, salt, and pepper.

3. Spread the vegetables evenly on the baking sheet and roast in the preheated oven for about 20-25 minutes until they are tender and slightly caramelized.

4. While the vegetables are roasting, prepare the couscous. In a saucepan, bring the vegetable broth to a boil. Stir in the couscous, cover, and remove from heat. Let it sit for about 5 minutes until the couscous absorbs the liquid.

5. Fluff the cooked couscous with a fork.

6. Once the roasted vegetables are done, combine them with the cooked couscous in a large bowl.

7. Toss everything together until well mixed.

8. Adjust the seasoning if needed.

9. Garnish with fresh parsley if desired.

10. Serve the roasted vegetable couscous warm or at room temperature.

TOMATO BASIL FARRO:

Preparation time: 10 minutes

Cooking time: 25 minutes

Servings: 4

Ingredients:

- 1 cup of farro

- 2 cups of vegetable broth

- 2 tablespoons of olive oil

- 2 cloves of garlic, minced

- 1 pint of cherry tomatoes, halved

- 1/4 cup of chopped fresh basil

- Salt and pepper to taste

- Grated Parmesan cheese for serving (optional)

Directions:

1. Rinse the farro under cold water.

2. In a saucepan, bring the vegetable broth to a boil. Add the rinsed farro, reduce the heat to low, cover, and simmer for about 20-25 minutes until the farro is tender and the broth is absorbed.

3. In a large skillet, heat the olive oil over medium heat.

4. Add the minced garlic to the skillet and sauté for 1-2 minutes until fragrant.

5. Add the halved cherry tomatoes to the skillet and cook for 3-4 minutes until they start to soften.

6. Stir in the cooked farro and chopped fresh basil. Mix well to combine all the ingredients.

7. Season with salt and pepper to taste.

8. Remove from heat and serve the tomato basil farro warm.

9. Optional: Sprinkle with grated Parmesan cheese before serving.

Enjoy your meal.

CREAMY AVOCADO PASTA:

Preparation time: 15 minutes

Cooking time: 10 minutes

Servings: 4

Ingredients:

- 8 ounces of spaghetti or your preferred pasta

- 2 ripe avocados, peeled and pitted

- 1/2 cup of fresh basil leaves

- 2 cloves of garlic, minced

- Juice of 1 lemon

- 2 tablespoons of extra virgin olive oil

- Salt and pepper to taste

- Optional toppings: cherry tomatoes, grated Parmesan cheese, red pepper flakes

Directions:

1. Cook the spaghetti according to the package instructions until al dente. Drain and set aside.

2. In a food processor or blender, combine the ripe avocados, basil leaves, minced garlic, lemon juice, extra virgin olive oil, salt, and pepper.

3. Blend until smooth and creamy.

4. In a large mixing bowl, toss the cooked spaghetti with the creamy avocado sauce until well coated.

5. Season with additional salt and pepper if needed.

6. Serve the creamy avocado pasta with optional toppings such as halved cherry tomatoes, grated Parmesan cheese, and red pepper flakes.

Greek Lemon Rice:

Preparation time: 5 minutes

Cooking time: 25 minutes

Servings: 4

Ingredients:

- 1 cup of long-grain white rice

- 2 cups of vegetable broth

- Juice of 1 lemon

- Zest of 1 lemon

- 2 tablespoons of olive oil

- 1 small onion, finely chopped

- 2 cloves of garlic, minced

- 1 teaspoon of dried oregano

- Salt and pepper to taste

- Chopped fresh parsley for garnish (optional)

Directions:

1. In a saucepan, heat the olive oil over medium heat.

2. Add the finely chopped onion to the saucepan and sauté for 3-4 minutes until translucent.

3. Stir in the minced garlic and dried oregano and cook for an additional minute.

4. Add the rice to the saucepan and stir to coat the grains with the onion and garlic mixture.

5. Pour in the vegetable broth, lemon juice, and lemon zest. Stir well.

6. Bring the mixture to a boil, then reduce the heat to low, cover, and simmer for about 15-20 minutes until the rice is cooked and the liquid is absorbed.

7. Fluff the cooked rice with a fork.

8. Season with salt and pepper to taste.

9. Garnish with chopped fresh parsley if desired.

10. Serve the Greek lemon rice hot.

BUTTERNUT SQUASH MAC AND CHEESE:

Preparation time: 15 minutes

Cooking time: 45 minutes

Servings: 6

Ingredients:

- 12 ounces of macaroni or your preferred pasta

- 4 cups of peeled and cubed butternut squash

- 2 tablespoons of butter

- 1 small onion, chopped

- 2 cloves of garlic, minced

- 2 cups of vegetable broth

- 1 cup of milk

- 2 cups of shredded cheddar cheese

- 1/4 cup of grated Parmesan cheese

- 1/2 teaspoon of dried thyme

- Salt and pepper to taste

- Optional toppings: breadcrumbs, chopped fresh parsley

Directions:

1. Cook the macaroni according to the package instructions until al dente. Drain and set aside.

2. Place the butternut squash cubes in a steamer basket and steam for about 10-15 minutes until tender.

3. In a large skillet, melt the butter over medium heat.

4. Add the chopped onion and minced garlic to the skillet and sauté for 3-4 minutes until the onion is translucent.

5. Add the steamed butternut squash to the skillet and mash it with a fork or potato masher until smooth.

6. Pour in the vegetable broth and milk. Stir well to combine.

7. Add the shredded cheddar cheese, grated Parmesan cheese, dried thyme, salt, and pepper to the skillet. Stir until the cheeses are melted and the sauce is smooth.

8. Add the cooked macaroni to the skillet and toss to coat the pasta with the butternut squash cheese sauce.

9. Preheat the oven to 375°F (190°C).

10. Transfer the mac and cheese mixture to a baking dish.

11. Optional: Sprinkle breadcrumbs on top of the mac and cheese for a crispy crust.

12. Bake in the preheated oven for about 20 minutes until the top is golden and bubbly.

13. Remove from the oven and let it cool for a few minutes before serving.

14. Garnish with chopped fresh parsley if desired.

Spinach and Artichoke Pasta:

Preparation time: 10 minutes

Cooking time: 20 minutes

Servings: 4

Ingredients:

- 8 ounces of penne or your preferred pasta

- 2 tablespoonsof olive oil

- 4 cloves of garlic, minced

- 1 can (14 ounces) of artichoke hearts, drained and chopped

- 4 cups of fresh spinach leaves

- 1 cup of heavy cream

- 1/2 cup of grated Parmesan cheese

- Salt and pepper to taste

- Optional toppings: red pepper flakes, grated Parmesan cheese

Directions:

1. Cook the penne according to the package instructions until al dente. Drain and set aside.

2. In a large skillet, heat the olive oil over medium heat.

3. Add the minced garlic to the skillet and sauté for 1-2 minutes until fragrant.

4. Add the chopped artichoke hearts to the skillet and cook for 3-4 minutes until they start to brown slightly.

5. Add the spinach leaves to the skillet and cook until wilted.

6. Pour in the heavy cream and stir well to combine.

7. Stir in the grated Parmesan cheese and continue cooking until the sauce thickens.

8. Season with salt and pepper to taste.

9. Add the cooked penne to the skillet and toss to coat the pasta with the spinach and artichoke sauce.

10. Cook for an additional 2-3 minutes until the pasta is heated through.

11. Optional: Sprinkle red pepper flakes and grated Parmesan cheese on top for added flavor and garnish.

12. Serve the spinach and artichoke pasta hot.

ROASTED VEGETABLE LASAGNA:

Preparation time: 30 minutes

Cooking time: 1 hour

Servings: 8-10

Ingredients:

- 12 lasagna noodles

- 2 cups of ricotta cheese

- 2 cups of shredded mozzarella cheese

- 1 cup of grated Parmesan cheese

- 2 cups of roasted vegetables (such as zucchini, bell peppers, eggplant, and mushrooms)

- 2 cups of marinara sauce

- 2 cloves of garlic, minced

- 1 teaspoon of dried basil

- 1 teaspoon of dried oregano

- Salt and pepper to taste

- Fresh basil leaves for garnish (optional)

Directions:

1. Preheat the oven to 375°F (190°C).

2. Cook the lasagna noodles according to the package instructions until al dente. Drain and set aside.

3. In a mixing bowl, combine the ricotta cheese, shredded mozzarella cheese, and grated Parmesan cheese. Mix well.

4. In a separate bowl, combine the roasted vegetables, minced garlic, dried basil, dried oregano, salt, and pepper. Toss to coat the vegetables with the seasonings.

5. Spread a thin layer of marinara sauce in the bottom of a baking dish.

6. Place a layer of cooked lasagna noodles on top of the sauce.

7. Spread a layer of the ricotta cheese mixture over the noodles.

8. Add a layer of the roasted vegetable mixture on top of the cheese.

9. Repeat these layers until all the ingredients are used, finishing with a layer of marinara sauce and shredded mozzarella cheese on top.

10. Cover the baking dish with foil and bake in the preheated oven for 45 minutes.

11. Remove the foil and bake for an additional 15 minutes until the cheese is bubbly and golden.

12. Let the lasagna cool for a few minutes before serving.

13. Garnish with fresh basil leaves if desired.

14. Serve the roasted vegetable lasagna warm.

Quinoa and Black Bean Salad:

Preparation time: 15 minutes

Cooking time: 15 minutes

Servings: 4

Ingredients:

- 1 cup of quinoa

- 2 cups of vegetable broth or water

- 1 can (15 ounces) of black beans, rinsed and drained

- 1 cup of cherry tomatoes, halved

- 1 small red bell pepper, diced

- 1 small cucumber, diced

- 1/4 cup of red onion, finely chopped

- 1/4 cup of fresh cilantro, chopped

- Juice of 1 lime

- 2 tablespoons of extra virgin olive oil

- 1 teaspoon of ground cumin

- Salt and pepper to taste

- Optional toppings: avocado slices, crumbled feta cheese

Directions:

1. Rinse the quinoa under cold water to remove any bitterness.

2. In a saucepan, bring the vegetable broth or water to a boil.

3. Add the quinoa to the boiling liquid, reduce the heat to low, cover, and simmer for about 15 minutes until the quinoa is cooked and the liquid is absorbed.

4. Remove the saucepan from the heat and let the quinoa cool for a few minutes.

5. In a large mixing bowl, combine the cooked quinoa, black beans, cherry tomatoes, red bell pepper, cucumber, red onion, and cilantro.

6. In a small bowl, whisk together the lime juice, extra virgin olive oil, ground cumin, salt, and pepper.

7. Pour the dressing over the quinoa and black bean mixture. Toss well to combine.

8. Adjust the seasoning if needed.

9. Optional: Top the salad with avocado slices and crumbled feta cheese for added flavor and garnish.

10. Serve the quinoa and black bean salad chilled or at room temperature.

Mushroom and Spinach Linguine:

Preparation time: 10 minutes

Cooking time: 20 minutes

Servings: 4

Ingredients:

- 8 ounces of linguine or your preferred pasta

- 2 tablespoons of olive oil

- 1 small onion, chopped

- 2 cloves of garlic, minced

- 8 ounces of mushrooms, sliced

- 4 cups of fresh spinach leaves

- 1 cup of vegetable broth

- 1/4 cup of grated Parmesan cheese

- Salt and pepper to taste

- Optional toppings: chopped fresh parsley, grated Parmesan cheese

Directions:

1. Cook the linguine according to the package instructions until al dente. Drain and set aside.

2. In a large skillet, heat the olive oil over medium heat.

3. Add the chopped onion to the skillet and sauté for 3-4 minutes until translucent.

4. Stir in the minced garlic and cook for an additional minute.

5. Add the sliced mushrooms to the skillet and cook for 5-7 minutes until they release their moisture and start to brown.

6. Add the fresh spinach leaves to the skillet and cook until wilted.

7. Pour in the vegetable broth and bring the mixture to a simmer.

8. Reduce the heat to low and stir in the grated Parmesan cheese.

9. Season with salt and pepper to taste.

10. Add the cooked linguine to the skillet and toss to coat the pasta with the mushroom and spinach sauce.

11. Cook for an additional 2-3 minutes until the pasta is heated through and well coated.

12. Optional: Sprinkle chopped fresh parsley and grated Parmesan cheese on top for added flavor and garnish.

13. Serve the mushroom and spinach linguine hot.

RATATOUILLE PASTA:

Preparation time: 15 minutes

Cooking time: 25 minutes

Servings: 4

Ingredients:

- 8 ounces of penne or your preferred pasta

- 2 tablespoons of olive oil

- 1 small onion, diced

- 2 cloves of garlic, minced

- 1 small eggplant, diced

- 1 small zucchini, diced

- 1 small yellow bell pepper, diced

- 1 small red bell pepper, diced

- 1 can (14 ounces) of diced tomatoes

- 1 teaspoon of dried basil

- 1 teaspoon of dried oregano

- Salt and pepper to taste

- Fresh basil leaves for garnish (optional)

Directions:

1. Cook the penne according to the package instructions until al dente. Drain and set aside.

2. In a large skillet, heat the olive oil over medium heat.

3. Add the diced onion to the skillet and sauté for 3-4 minutes until translucent.

4. Stir in the minced garlic and cook for an additional minute.

5. Add the diced eggplant, zucchini, yellow bell pepper, and red bell pepper to the skillet. Stir well to coat the vegetables with the oil and onion mixture.

6. Cook for about 10 minutes, stirring occasionally,until the vegetables are tender.

7. Pour in the diced tomatoes, including the liquid from the can.

8. Add the dried basil, dried oregano, salt, and pepper to the skillet. Stir to combine.

9. Simmer the mixture for about 10 minutes, allowing the flavors to blend together.

10. Add the cooked penne to the skillet and toss to coat the pasta with the ratatouille sauce.

11. Cook for an additional 2-3 minutes until the pasta is heated through.

12. Optional: Garnish with fresh basil leaves for added flavor and presentation.

13. Serve the ratatouille pasta hot.

LEMON HERB QUINOA:

Preparation time: 10 minutes

Cooking time: 20 minutes

Servings: 4

Ingredients:

- 1 cup of quinoa

- 2 cups of vegetable broth or water

- Zest and juice of 1 lemon

- 2 tablespoons of chopped fresh herbs (such as parsley, basil, or cilantro)

- 2 tablespoons of extra virgin olive oil

- Salt and pepper to taste

- Optional toppings: lemon wedges, chopped fresh herbs

Directions:

1. Rinse the quinoa under cold water to remove any bitterness.

2. In a saucepan, bring the vegetable broth or water to a boil.

3. Add the quinoa to the boiling liquid, reduce the heat to low, cover, and simmer for about 15 minutes until the quinoa is cooked and the liquid is absorbed.

4. Remove the saucepan from the heat and let the quinoa cool for a few minutes.

5. In a mixing bowl, combine the cooked quinoa, lemon zest, lemon juice, chopped fresh herbs, extra virgin olive oil, salt, and pepper.

6. Toss the ingredients together until well combined.

7. Adjust the seasoning if needed.

8. Optional: Serve the lemon herb quinoa with lemon wedges and garnish with additional chopped fresh herbs for added flavor and presentation.

9. Serve the lemon herb quinoa warm or at room temperature.

<h1 style="text-align:center">Vegetable Biryani:</h1>

Preparation time: 20 minutes

Cooking time: 40 minutes

Servings: 4

Ingredients:

- 1 cup of basmati rice

- 2 cups of water

- 2 tablespoons of ghee or vegetable oil

- 1 medium onion, thinly sliced

- 2 cloves of garlic, minced

- 1-inch piece of ginger, grated

- 1 small green chili, finely chopped (optional, adjust according to spice preference)

- 1 teaspoon of cumin seeds

- 1 teaspoon of ground coriander

- 1/2 teaspoon of ground turmeric

- 1/2 teaspoon of ground cinnamon

- 1/4 teaspoon of ground cardamom

- 1 cup of mixed vegetables (such as carrots, peas, bell peppers, and cauliflower), diced

- 1/4 cup of golden raisins

- 1/4 cup of cashews

- Salt to taste

- Fresh cilantro leaves for garnish

Directions:

1. Rinse the basmati rice under cold water until the water runs clear.

2. In a saucepan, bring the water to a boil. Add the rinsed rice and cook until it is 70-80% cooked (about 8-10 minutes). The rice should be slightly undercooked as it will continue cooking later.

3. Drain the rice and set it aside.

4. In a large skillet or pot, heat the ghee or vegetable oil over medium heat.

5. Add the sliced onion and sauté until golden brown and caramelized.

6. Stir in the minced garlic, grated ginger, and chopped green chili. Cook for an additional minute.

7. Add the cumin seeds, ground coriander, ground turmeric, ground cinnamon, and ground cardamom to the skillet. Stir well to coat the onions and spices.

8. Add the diced mixed vegetables to the skillet and sauté for 5-7 minutes until they are slightly tender.

9. Stir in the golden raisins and cashews.

10. Gently fold in the partially cooked rice and mix everything together.

11. Season with salt to taste.

12. Reduce the heat to low, cover the skillet or pot, and let the biryani cook for about 15-20 minutes until the rice is fully cooked and the flavors have melded together.

13. Optional: Garnish the vegetable biryani with fresh cilantro leaves for added flavor and presentation.

14. Serve the vegetable biryani hot as a main course or as a side dish with raita (yogurt sauce) or pickle.

Chapter 5

Soups & Stews

Tomato Basil Soup:

Preparation time: 10 minutes

Cooking time: 30 minutes

Servings: 4

Ingredients:

- 2 tablespoons of olive oil

- 1 small onion, chopped

- 2 cloves of garlic, minced

- 1 can (28 ounces) of crushed tomatoes

- 1 cup of vegetable broth

- 1/4 cup of fresh basil leaves, chopped

- 1 teaspoon of dried oregano

- 1/2 teaspoon of sugar

- Salt and pepper to taste

- Optional toppings: fresh basil leaves, grated Parmesan cheese, croutons

Directions:

1. In a large saucepan, heat the olive oil over medium heat.

2. Add the chopped onion to the saucepan and sauté until it becomes translucent.

3. Stir in the minced garlic and cook for an additional minute.

4. Add the crushed tomatoes, vegetable broth, chopped basil leaves, dried oregano, sugar, salt, and pepper to the saucepan. Stir well to combine.

5. Bring the mixture to a boil, then reduce the heat to low and simmer for about 20 minutes, allowing the flavors to meld together.

6. Use an immersion blender or a countertop blender to blend the soup until smooth.

7. Adjust the seasoning if needed.

8. Optional: Serve the tomato basil soup garnished with fresh basil leaves, grated Parmesan cheese, and croutons for added flavor and texture.

9. Serve the soup hot.

Lentil Soup with Vegetables:

Preparation time: 10 minutes

Cooking time: 40 minutes

Servings: 4

Ingredients:

- 1 cup of dried lentils (green or brown), rinsed and drained

- 4 cups of vegetable broth

- 1 tablespoon of olive oil

- 1 small onion, chopped

- 2 cloves of garlic, minced

- 2 carrots, diced

- 2 celery stalks, diced

- 1 small zucchini, diced

- 1 can (14 ounces) of diced tomatoes

- 1 teaspoon of ground cumin

- 1 teaspoon of ground coriander

- 1/2 teaspoon of smoked paprika

- Salt and pepper to taste

- Fresh parsley leaves for garnish

Directions:

1. In a large pot, combine the rinsed lentils and vegetable broth. Bring the mixture to a boil over medium heat.

2. Reduce the heat to low and simmer, partially covered, for about 20-25 minutes until the lentils are tender.

3. In a separate skillet, heat the olive oil over medium heat.

4. Add the chopped onion to the skillet and sauté until it becomes translucent.

5. Stir in the minced garlic and cook for an additional minute.

6. Add the diced carrots, celery, zucchini, diced tomatoes (including the liquid from the can), ground cumin, ground coriander, smoked paprika, salt, and pepper to the skillet. Stir well to combine.

7. Cook the vegetable mixture for about 10 minutes until the vegetables are tender.

8. Add the cooked lentils and their broth to the skillet with the vegetables. Stir to combine.

9. Simmer the soup for an additional 5 minutes to allow the flavors to meld together.

10. Adjust the seasoning if needed.

11. Optional: Garnish the lentil soup with fresh parsley leaves for added flavor and presentation.

12. Serve the soup hot.

MINESTRONE SOUP:

Preparation time: 15 minutes

Cooking time: 35 minutes

Servings: 4

Ingredients:

- 2 tablespoons of olive oil

- 1 small onion, chopped

- 2 cloves of garlic, minced

- 2 carrots, diced

- 2 celery stalks, diced

- 1 small zucchini, diced

- 1 small yellow squash, diced

- 1 can (14 ounces) of diced tomatoes

- 4 cups of vegetable broth

- 1 teaspoon of dried basil

- 1 teaspoon of dried oregano

- 1/2 teaspoon of dried thyme

- 1/2 cup of small pasta (such as macaroni or small shells)

- 1 can (15 ounces) of kidney beans, rinsed and drained

- Salt and pepper to taste

- Fresh parsley leaves for garnish

- Grated Parmesan cheese for garnish (optional)

Directions:

1. In a large pot, heat the olive oil over medium heat.

2. Add the chopped onion to the pot and sauté until it becomes translucent.

3. Stir in the minced garlic and cook for an additional minute.

4. Add the diced carrots, celery, zucchini, yellow squash, diced tomatoes (including the liquid from the can), vegetable broth, dried basil, dried oregano, and dried thyme to the pot. Stir well to combine.

5. Bring the mixture to aboil, then reduce the heat to low and simmer for about 20 minutes, allowing the flavors to meld together.

6. In a separate pot, cook the small pasta according to the package instructions until al dente. Drain and set aside.

7. Add the cooked pasta and kidney beans to the pot with the vegetable mixture. Stir to combine.

8. Simmer the soup for an additional 5 minutes to heat through.

9. Adjust the seasoning with salt and pepper to taste.

10. Optional: Garnish the minestrone soup with fresh parsley leaves and grated Parmesan cheese for added flavor and presentation.

11. Serve the soup hot.

Creamy Broccoli Soup:

Preparation time: 15 minutes

Cooking time: 25 minutes

Servings: 4

Ingredients:

- 2 tablespoons of butter

- 1 small onion, chopped

- 2 cloves of garlic, minced

- 4 cups of broccoli florets

- 3 cups of vegetable broth

- 1 cup of milk

- 1/2 cup of heavy cream

- Salt and pepper to taste

- Optional toppings: grated cheddar cheese, croutons, chopped chives

Directions:

1. In a large pot, melt the butter over medium heat.

2. Add the chopped onion to the pot and sauté until it becomes translucent.

3. Stir in the minced garlic and cook for an additional minute.

4. Add the broccoli florets and vegetable broth to the pot. Bring the mixture to a boil, then reduce the heat to low and simmer for about 15 minutes until the broccoli is tender.

5. Use an immersion blender or a countertop blender to puree the soup until smooth.

6. Return the soup to the pot and stir in the milk and heavy cream.

7. Season with salt and pepper to taste.

8. Cook the soup for an additional 5 minutes to heat through.

9. Optional: Serve the creamy broccoli soup garnished with grated cheddar cheese, croutons, and chopped chives for added flavor and texture.

10. Serve the soup hot.

Moroccan Vegetable Stew:

Preparation time: 15 minutes

Cooking time: 40 minutes

Servings: 4

Ingredients:

- 2 tablespoons of olive oil

- 1 small onion, chopped

- 2 cloves of garlic, minced

- 2 carrots, diced

- 1 small eggplant, diced

- 1 zucchini, diced

- 1 red bell pepper, diced

- 1 can (14 ounces) of diced tomatoes

- 2 cups of vegetable broth

- 1 teaspoon of ground cumin

- 1 teaspoon of ground coriander

- 1/2 teaspoon of ground cinnamon

- 1/2 teaspoon of paprika

- 1/4 teaspoon of cayenne pepper (optional, for heat)

- Salt and pepper to taste

- Fresh cilantro leaves for garnish

Directions:

1. In a large pot, heat the olive oil over medium heat.

2. Add the chopped onion to the pot and sauté until it becomes translucent.

3. Stir in the minced garlic and cook for an additional minute.

4. Add the diced carrots, eggplant, zucchini, red bell pepper, diced tomatoes (including the liquid from the can), vegetable broth, ground cumin, ground coriander, ground cinnamon, paprika, cayenne pepper (if using), salt, and pepper to the pot. Stir well to combine.

5. Bring the mixture to a boil, then reduce the heat to low and simmer for about 30 minutes until the vegetables are tender.

6. Adjust the seasoning with salt and pepper to taste.

7. Optional: Garnish the Moroccan vegetable stew with fresh cilantro leaves for added flavor and presentation.

8. Serve the stew hot.

Enjoy your soups and stews

BUTTERNUT SQUASH SOUP:

Preparation time: 15 minutes

Cooking time: 45 minutes

Servings: 4

Ingredients:

- 1 medium butternut squash, peeled, seeded, and cut into cubes

- 1 tablespoon of olive oil

- 1 small onion, chopped

- 2 cloves of garlic, minced

- 4 cups of vegetable broth

- 1 teaspoon of ground cumin

- 1/2 teaspoon of ground cinnamon

- 1/4 teaspoon of ground nutmeg

- Salt and pepper to taste

- Optional toppings: roasted pumpkin seeds, sour cream, chopped fresh parsley

Directions:

1. Preheat the oven to 400°F (200°C).

2. Place the butternut squash cubes on a baking sheet and drizzle with olive oil. Toss to coat evenly.

3. Roast the butternut squash in the preheated oven for about 25-30 minutes, or until it is tender and slightly caramelized.

4. In a large pot, heat the olive oil over medium heat.

5. Add the chopped onion to the pot and sauté until it becomes translucent.

6. Stir in the minced garlic and cook for an additional minute.

7. Add the roasted butternut squash cubes, vegetable broth, ground cumin, ground cinnamon, ground nutmeg, salt, and pepper to the pot. Stir well to combine.

8. Bring the mixture to a boil, then reduce the heat to low and simmer for about 15 minutes to allow the flavors to meld together.

9. Use an immersion blender or a countertop blender to puree the soup until smooth.

10. Adjust the seasoning with salt and pepper to taste.

11. Optional: Serve the butternut squash soup garnished with roasted pumpkin seeds, a dollop of sour cream, and chopped fresh parsley for added flavor and texture.

12. Serve the soup hot.

SPINACH AND WHITE BEAN SOUP:

Preparation time: 10 minutes

Cooking time: 25 minutes

Servings: 4

Ingredients:

- 2 tablespoons of olive oil

- 1 small onion, chopped

- 2 cloves of garlic, minced

- 4 cups of vegetable broth

- 1 can (15 ounces) of white beans, rinsed and drained

- 4 cups of fresh spinach leaves

- 1 teaspoon of dried thyme

- Salt and pepper to taste

- Optional toppings: grated Parmesan cheese, lemon wedges

Directions:

1. In a large pot, heat the olive oil over medium heat.

2. Add the chopped onion to the pot and sauté until it becomes translucent.

3. Stir in the minced garlic and cook for an additional minute.

4. Add the vegetable broth, white beans, fresh spinach leaves, dried thyme, salt, and pepper to the pot. Stir well to combine.

5. Bring the mixture to a boil, then reduce the heat to low and simmer for about 15-20 minutes to allow the flavors to meld together and the spinach to wilt.

6. Adjust the seasoning with salt and pepper to taste.

7. Optional: Serve the spinach and white bean soup garnished with grated Parmesan cheese and a squeeze of lemon juice for added flavor and freshness.

8. Serve the soup hot.

SWEET POTATO AND LENTIL SOUP:

Preparation time: 15 minutes

Cooking time: 35 minutes

Servings: 4

Ingredients:

- 2 tablespoons of olive oil

- 1 small onion, chopped

- 2 cloves of garlic, minced

- 2 medium sweet potatoes, peeled and diced

- 1 cup of dried red lentils, rinsed and drained

- 4 cups of vegetable broth

- 1 teaspoon of ground cumin

- 1/2 teaspoon of ground coriander

- 1/2 teaspoon of smoked paprika

- Salt and pepper to taste

- Optional toppings: Greek yogurt, chopped fresh cilantro

Directions:

1. In a large pot, heat the olive oil over medium heat.

2. Add the chopped onion to the pot and sauté until it becomes translucent.

3. Stir in the minced garlic and cook for an additional minute.

4. Add the diced sweet potatoes, red lentils, vegetable broth, ground cumin, ground coriander, smoked paprika, salt, and pepper to the pot. Stir well to combine.

5. Bring the mixture to a boil, then reduce the heat to low and simmer for about 20-25 minutes until the sweet potatoes and lentils are tender.

6. Use an immersion blender or a countertop blender to puree about half of the soup, leaving some chunks for texture.

7. Adjust the seasoning with salt and pepper to taste.

8. Optional: Serve the sweet potato and lentil soup garnished with a dollop of Greek yogurt and chopped fresh cilantro for added creaminess and freshness.

9. Serve the soup hotMexican Black Bean Soup:

Preparation time: 10 minutes

Cooking time: 30 minutes

Servings: 4

Ingredients:

- 2 tablespoons of olive oil

- 1 small onion, chopped

- 2 cloves of garlic, minced

- 1 red bell pepper, diced

- 1 jalapeno pepper, seeded and minced (optional)

- 2 teaspoons of ground cumin

- 1 teaspoon of chili powder

- 1 can (15 ounces) of black beans, rinsed and drained

- 1 can (14.5 ounces) of diced tomatoes

- 3 cups of vegetable broth

- Juice of 1 lime

- Salt and pepper to taste

- Optional toppings: chopped fresh cilantro, diced avocado, shredded cheese, tortilla chips

Directions:

1. In a large pot, heat the olive oil over medium heat.

2. Add the chopped onion, minced garlic, diced red bell pepper, and minced jalapeno pepper (if using) to the pot. Sauté until the vegetables are tender.

3. Stir in the ground cumin and chili powder, and cook for an additional minute to toast the spices.

4. Add the black beans, diced tomatoes (with their juices), vegetable broth, and lime juice to the pot. Stir well to combine.

5. Bring the mixture to a boil, then reduce the heat to low and simmer for about 15-20 minutes to allow the flavors to meld together.

6. Use an immersion blender or a countertop blender to puree about half of the soup, leaving some beans and vegetables for texture.

7. Adjust the seasoning with salt and pepper to taste.

8. Optional: Serve the Mexican black bean soup garnished with chopped fresh cilantro, diced avocado, shredded cheese, and tortilla chips for added flavor and crunch.

9. Serve the soup hot.

Vegetarian Chili:

Preparation time: 15 minutes

Cooking time: 1 hour 15 minutes

Servings: 6

Ingredients:

- 2 tablespoons of olive oil

- 1 large onion, chopped

- 2 cloves of garlic, minced

- 1 red bell pepper, diced

- 1 green bell pepper, diced

- 1 jalapeno pepper, seeded and minced (optional)

- 2 carrots, diced

- 2 celery stalks, diced

- 1 zucchini, diced

- 1 can (15 ounces) of kidney beans, rinsed and drained

- 1 can (15 ounces) of black beans, rinsed and drained

- 1 can (15 ounces) of diced tomatoes

- 1 can (6 ounces) of tomato paste

- 2 cups of vegetable broth

- 2 tablespoons of chili powder

- 1 teaspoon of ground cumin

- 1 teaspoon of dried oregano

- Salt and pepper to taste

- Optional toppings: shredded cheese, diced avocado, sour cream, chopped green onions

Directions:

1. In a large pot, heat the olive oil over medium heat.

2. Add the chopped onion, minced garlic, diced red bell pepper, diced green bell pepper, and minced jalapeno pepper (if using) to the pot. Sauté until the vegetables are tender.

3. Add the diced carrots, diced celery, and diced zucchini to the pot. Cook for an additional 5 minutes.

4. Stir in the kidney beans, black beans, diced tomatoes (with their juices), tomato paste, vegetable broth, chili powder, ground cumin, dried oregano, salt, and pepper. Stir well to combine.

5. Bring the mixture to a boil, then reduce the heat to low and simmer for about 1 hour to allow the flavors to develop and the chili to thicken. Stir occasionally.

6. Adjust the seasoning with salt and pepper to taste.

7. Optional: Serve the vegetarian chili garnished with shredded cheese, diced avocado, a dollop of sour cream, and chopped green onions for added flavor and creaminess.

8. Serve the chili hot.

Enjoy your delicious soups and chili

CREAMY CAULIFLOWER SOUP:

Preparation time: 10 minutes

Cooking time: 30 minutes

Servings: 4

Ingredients:

- 1 large head of cauliflower, chopped into florets

- 2 tablespoons of butter or olive oil

- 1 medium onion, chopped

- 2 cloves of garlic, minced

- 4 cups of vegetable broth

- 1 cup of milk (or dairy-free milk for a vegan option)

- Salt and pepper to taste

- Optional toppings: chopped fresh chives, grated Parmesan cheese

Directions:

1. In a large pot, melt the butter or heat the olive oil over medium heat.

2. Add the chopped onion and minced garlic to the pot. Sauté until the onion becomes translucent.

3. Add the cauliflower florets to the pot and stir well to coat them with the onion and garlic mixture.

4. Pour in the vegetable broth and bring the mixture to a boil.

5. Reduce the heat to low, cover the pot, and simmer for about 20-25 minutes, or until the cauliflower is tender.

6. Use an immersion blender or a countertop blender to puree the soup until smooth and creamy.

7. Return the soup to the pot and stir in the milk. Heat the soup over low heat until warmed through.

8. Season with salt and pepper to taste.

9. Optional: Serve the creamy cauliflower soup garnished with chopped fresh chives and grated Parmesan cheese for added flavor and texture.

10. Serve the soup hot.

QUINOA AND VEGETABLE STEW:

Preparation time: 15 minutes

Cooking time: 30 minutes

Servings: 4

Ingredients:

- 1 tablespoon of olive oil

- 1 small onion, chopped

- 2 cloves of garlic, minced

- 2 carrots, diced

- 2 celery stalks, diced

- 1 red bell pepper, diced

- 1 zucchini, diced

- 1 cup of cooked quinoa

- 1 can (15 ounces) of diced tomatoes

- 4 cups of vegetable broth

- 1 teaspoon of dried thyme

- 1 teaspoon of dried oregano

- Salt and pepper to taste

- Optional toppings: chopped fresh parsley, grated Parmesan cheese

Directions:

1. In a large pot, heat the olive oil over medium heat.

2. Add the chopped onion and minced garlic to the pot. Sauté until the onion becomes translucent.

3. Add the diced carrots, diced celery, diced red bell pepper, and diced zucchini to the pot. Cook for about 5 minutes until the vegetables start to soften.

4. Stir in the cooked quinoa, diced tomatoes (with their juices), vegetable broth, dried thyme, dried oregano, salt, and pepper. Stir well to combine.

5. Bring the mixture to a boil, then reduce the heat to low and simmer for about 20-25 minutes to allow the flavors to meld together.

6. Adjust the seasoning with salt and pepper to taste.

7. Optional: Serve the quinoa and vegetable stew garnished with chopped fresh parsley and grated Parmesan cheese for added flavor and freshness.

8. Serve the stew hot.

Carrot and Ginger Soup:

Preparation time: 10 minutes

Cooking time: 25 minutes

Servings: 4

Ingredients:

- 2 tablespoons of olive oil

- 1 small onion, chopped

- 2 cloves of garlic, minced

- 1 pound of carrots, peeled and chopped

- 1 tablespoon of grated fresh ginger

- 4 cups of vegetable broth

- 1 can (14 ounces) of coconut milk

- Salt and pepper to taste

- Optional toppings: chopped fresh cilantro, toasted pumpkin seeds

Directions:

1. In a large pot, heat the olive oil over medium heat.

2. Add the chopped onion and minced garlic to the pot. Sauté until the onion becomes translucent.

3. Add the chopped carrots and grated ginger to the pot. Cook for about 5 minutes until the carrots start to soften.

4. Pour in the vegetable broth and bring the mixture to a boil.

5. Reduce the heat to low, cover the pot, and simmer for about 15-20 minutes, or until the carrots are tender.

6. Use an immersion blender or a countertop blender to puree the soup until smooth.

7. Return the soup to the pot and stir in the coconut milk. Heat the soup over low heat until warmed through.

8. Season with salt and pepper to taste.

9. Optional: Serve the carrot and ginger soup garnished with chopped fresh cilantro and toasted pumpkin seeds for added flavor and crunch.

10. Serve the soup hot.

SPINACH AND TOMATO SOUP:

Preparation time: 10 minutes

Cooking time: 25 minutes

Servings: 4

Ingredients:

- 2 tablespoons of olive oil

- 1 small onion, chopped

- 2 cloves of garlic, minced

- 1 can (14 ounces) of diced tomatoes

- 4 cups of vegetable broth

- 4 cups of fresh spinach leaves

- 1 teaspoon of dried basil

- 1 teaspoon of dried oregano

- Salt and pepper to taste

- Optional toppings: grated Parmesan cheese, croutons

Directions:

1. In a large pot, heat the olive oil over medium heat.

2. Add the chopped onion and minced garlic to the pot. Sauté until the onion becomes translucent.

3. Add the diced tomatoes (with their juices) to the pot and cook for about 5 minutes to allow the flavors to meld together.

4. Pour in the vegetable broth and bring the mixture to a boil.

5. Reduce the heat to low and add the fresh spinach leaves to the pot. Cook for a few minutes until the spinach wilts.

6. Stir in the dried basil, dried oregano, salt, and pepper. Adjust the seasoning according to your taste.

7. Optional: Use an immersion blender or a countertop blender to puree the soup partially for a chunky texture, or puree completely for a smoother consistency.

8. Serve the spinach and tomato soup hot.

9. Optional: Top the soup with grated Parmesan cheese and croutons for added flavor and texture.

CREAMY MUSHROOM SOUP:

Preparation time: 10 minutes

Cooking time: 25 minutes

Servings: 4

Ingredients:

- 2 tablespoons of butter or olive oil

- 1 small onion, chopped

- 2 cloves of garlic, minced

- 1 pound of mushrooms, sliced

- 4 cups of vegetable broth

- 1 cup of heavy cream (or dairy-free cream for a vegan option)

- Salt and pepper to taste

- Optional toppings: chopped fresh parsley, sautéed mushrooms

Directions:

1. In a large pot, melt the butter or heat the olive oil over medium heat.

2. Add the chopped onion and minced garlic to the pot. Sauté until the onion becomes translucent.

3. Add the sliced mushrooms to the pot and cook for about 5 minutes until they release their moisture and start to brown.

4. Pour in the vegetable broth and bring the mixture to a boil.

5. Reduce the heat to low and simmer for about 15-20 minutes to allow the flavors to develop.

6. Use an immersion blender or a countertop blender to puree the soup until smooth.

7. Return the soup to the pot and stir in the heavy cream. Heat the soup over low heat until warmed through.

8. Season with salt and pepper to taste.

9. Optional: Serve the creamy mushroom soup garnished with chopped fresh parsley and sautéed mushrooms for added flavor and presentation.

10. Serve the soup hot.

CHICKPEA AND VEGETABLE STEW:

Preparation time: 15 minutes

Cooking time: 30 minutes

Servings: 4

Ingredients:

- 2 tablespoons of olive oil

- 1 small onion, chopped

- 2 cloves of garlic, minced

- 2 carrots, diced

- 2 celery stalks, diced

- 1 red bell pepper, diced

- 1 zucchini, diced

- 1 can (15 ounces) of chickpeas, drained and rinsed

- 1 can (14 ounces) of diced tomatoes

- 4 cups of vegetable broth

- 1 teaspoon of ground cumin

- 1 teaspoon of paprika

- Salt and pepper to taste

- Optional toppings: chopped fresh parsley, lemon wedges

Directions:

1. In a large pot, heat the olive oil over medium heat.

2. Add the chopped onion and minced garlic to the pot. Sauté until the onion becomes translucent.

3. Add the diced carrots, diced celery, diced red bell pepper, and diced zucchini to the pot. Cook for about 5 minutes until the vegetables start to soften.

4. Stir in the drained and rinsed chickpeas, diced tomatoes (with their juices), vegetable broth, ground cumin, paprika, salt, and pepper. Stir well to combine.

5. Bring the mixture to a boil, then reduce the heat to low and simmer for about 20-25 minutes to allow the flavors to meld together.

6. Adjust the seasoning with salt and pepper to taste.

7. Optional: Serve the chickpea and vegetable stew garnished with chopped fresh parsley and lemon wedges for added freshness and tanginess.

8. Serve the stew hot.

ROASTED RED PEPPER SOUP:

Preparation time: 15 minutes

Cooking time: 40 minutes

Servings: 4

Ingredients:

- 3 red bell peppers

- 2 tablespoons of olive oil

- 1 small onion, chopped

- 2 cloves of garlic, minced

- 1 can (14 ounces) of diced tomatoes

- 4 cups of vegetable broth

- 1 teaspoon of smoked paprika

- 1/2 teaspoon of dried thyme

- Salt and pepper to taste

- Optional toppings: Greek yogurt, chopped fresh basil

Directions:

1. Preheat the oven to 400°F (200°C).

2. Place the red bell peppers on a baking sheet and roast them in the preheated oven for about 20-25 minutes, or until the skins are charred and blistered.

3. Remove the peppers from the oven and transfer them to a bowl. Cover the bowl with plastic wrap and let the peppers steam for about 10 minutes.

4. Once the peppers are cool enough to handle, remove the skins, seeds, and stems. Chop the roasted peppers and set them aside.

5. In a large pot, heat the olive oil over medium heat.

6. Add the chopped onion and minced garlic to the pot. Sauté until the onion becomes translucent.

7. Stir in the chopped roasted peppers, diced tomatoes (with their juices), vegetable broth, smoked paprika, dried thyme, salt, and pepper. Stir well to combine.

8. Bring the mixture to a boil, then reduce the heat to low and simmer for about 15-20 minutes to allow the flavors to develop.

9. Use an immersion blender or a countertop blender to puree the soup until smooth.

10. Return the soup to the pot and heat it over low heat until warmed through.

11. Season with salt and pepper to taste.

12. Optional: Serve the roasted red pepper soup garnished with a dollop of Greek yogurt and chopped fresh basil for added creaminess and freshness.

13. Serve the soup hot.

Potato Leek Soup:

Preparation time: 15 minutes

Cooking time: 30 minutes

Servings: 4

Ingredients:

- 2 tablespoons of butter or olive oil

- 2 leeks, white and light green parts only, cleaned and thinly sliced

- 2 cloves of garlic, minced

- 4 cups of vegetable broth

- 4 medium-sized potatoes, peeled and diced

- 1 cup of milk (or dairy-free milk for a vegan option)

- Salt and pepper to taste

- Optional toppings: chopped fresh chives, crispy bacon bits

Directions:

1. In a large pot, melt the butter or heat the olive oil over medium heat.

2. Add the sliced leeks and minced garlic to the pot. Sauté until the leeks become soft and fragrant.

3. Pour in the vegetable broth and add the diced potatoes to the pot. Bring the mixture to a boil.

4. Reduce the heat to low, cover the pot, and simmer for about 20-25 minutes, or until the potatoes are tender.

5. Use an immersion blender or a countertop blender to puree the soup until smooth and creamy6. Return the soup to the pot and stir in the milk. Heat the soup over low heat until warmed through.

7. Season with salt and pepper to taste.

8. Optional: Serve the potato leek soup garnished with chopped fresh chives and crispy bacon bits for added flavor and texture.

9. Serve the soup hot.

Thai Coconut Curry Soup:

Preparation time: 15 minutes

Cooking time: 25 minutes

Servings: 4

Ingredients:

- 1 tablespoon of vegetable oil

- 1 small onion, chopped

- 2 cloves of garlic, minced

- 1 tablespoon of Thai red curry paste (adjust according to your spice preference)

- 1 can (14 ounces) of coconut milk

- 4 cups of vegetable broth

- 1 red bell pepper, thinly sliced

- 1 zucchini, diced

- 8 ounces of mushrooms, sliced

- 1 cup of fresh or frozen peas

- 1 tablespoon of soy sauce or tamari

- 1 tablespoon of lime juice

- Salt and pepper to taste

- Fresh cilantro for garnish

Directions:

1. In a large pot, heat the vegetable oil over medium heat.

2. Add the chopped onion and minced garlic to the pot. Sauté until the onion becomes translucent.

3. Stir in the Thai red curry paste and cook for about 1 minute to release its flavors.

4. Pour in the coconut milk and vegetable broth. Stir well to combine.

5. Add the sliced red bell pepper, diced zucchini, sliced mushrooms, and peas to the pot. Bring the mixture to a boil.

6. Reduce the heat to low and simmer for about 15-20 minutes, or until the vegetables are cooked to your liking.

7. Stir in the soy sauce or tamari and lime juice. Season with salt and pepper to taste.

8. Optional: Serve the Thai coconut curry soup garnished with fresh cilantro for added freshness and aroma.

9. Serve the soup hot.

SPINACH AND LENTIL STEW:

Preparation time: 15 minutes

Cooking time: 30 minutes

Servings: 4

Ingredients:

- 2 tablespoons of olive oil

- 1 small onion, chopped

- 2 cloves of garlic, minced

- 1 carrot, diced

- 1 celery stalk, diced

- 1 cup of dried green or brown lentils, rinsed

- 4 cups of vegetable broth

- 1 can (14 ounces) of diced tomatoes

- 2 teaspoons of ground cumin

- 1 teaspoon of paprika

- 1/2 teaspoon of ground turmeric

- 4 cups of fresh spinach leaves

- Salt and pepper to taste

- Optional toppings: Greek yogurt, chopped fresh parsley

Directions:

1. In a large pot, heat the olive oil over medium heat.

2. Add the chopped onion and minced garlic to the pot. Sauté until the onion becomes translucent.

3. Add the diced carrot and diced celery to the pot. Cook for about 5 minutes until the vegetables start to soften.

4. Stir in the rinsed lentils, vegetable broth, diced tomatoes (with their juices), ground cumin, paprika, and ground turmeric. Stir well to combine.

5. Bring the mixture to a boil, then reduce the heat to low and simmer for about 20-25 minutes, or until the lentils are tender.

6. Stir in the fresh spinach leaves and cook for an additional 2-3 minutes until the spinach wilts.

7. Season with salt and pepper to taste.

8. Optional: Serve the spinach and lentil stew garnished with a dollop of Greek yogurt and chopped fresh parsley for added creaminess and freshness.

9. Serve the stew hot.

Enjoy your delicious and comforting soups and stews

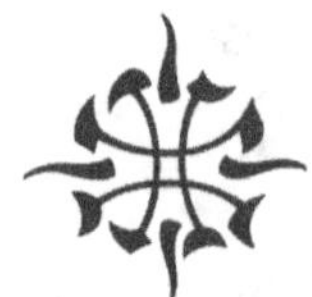

Chapter 6

Desserts & Baked Goods

Banana Bread with Walnuts:

Preparation time: 15 minutes

Baking time: 1 hour

Servings: 8

Ingredients:

- 2 cups of all-purpose flour

- 1 teaspoon of baking soda

- 1/2 teaspoon of salt

- 1/2 teaspoon of ground cinnamon

- 1/4 teaspoon of ground nutmeg

- 1/2 cup of unsalted butter, softened

- 1 cup of granulated sugar

- 2 large eggs

- 4 ripe bananas, mashed

- 1 teaspoon of vanilla extract

- 1/2 cup of chopped walnuts

Directions:

1. Preheat your oven to 350°F (175°C). Grease a 9x5-inch loaf pan.

2. In a medium bowl, whisk together the flour, baking soda, salt, cinnamon, and nutmeg. Set aside.

3. In a large bowl, cream together the softened butter and granulated sugar until light and fluffy.

4. Add the eggs, mashed bananas, and vanilla extract to the butter-sugar mixture. Mix well.

5. Gradually add the dry ingredients to the wet ingredients, mixing until just combined. Avoid overmixing.

6. Fold in the chopped walnuts.

7. Pour the batter into the prepared loaf pan and smooth the top with a spatula.

8. Bake in the preheated oven for about 60 minutes, or until a toothpick inserted into the center comes out clean.

9. Remove the banana bread from the oven and let it cool in the pan for 10 minutes.

10. Transfer the bread to a wire rack to cool completely before slicing.

11. Slice and serve the banana bread with walnuts.

BLUEBERRY OATMEAL MUFFINS:

Preparation time: 15 minutes

Baking time: 20-25 minutes

Servings: 12

Ingredients:

- 1 1/2 cups of all-purpose flour

- 1 cup of rolled oats

- 1/2 cup of granulated sugar

- 2 teaspoons of baking powder

- 1/2 teaspoon of baking soda

- 1/2 teaspoon of salt

- 1 cup of buttermilk

- 1/4 cup of unsalted butter, melted

- 1 large egg

- 1 teaspoon of vanilla extract

- 1 cup of fresh or frozen blueberries

Directions:

1. Preheat your oven to 375°F (190°C). Line a muffin tin with paper liners or grease the cups.

2. In a large bowl, combine the flour, oats, sugar, baking powder, baking soda, and salt.

3. In a separate bowl, whisk together the buttermilk, melted butter, egg, and vanilla extract.

4. Pour the wet ingredients into the dry ingredients and stir until just combined. Do not overmix.

5. Gently fold in the blueberries.

6. Divide the batter evenly among the muffin cups, filling each about two-thirds full.

7. Bake in the preheated oven for 20-25 minutes, or until a toothpick inserted into the center of a muffin comes out clean.

8. Remove the muffins from the oven and let them cool in the tin for a few minutes before transferring to a wire rack to cool completely.

9. Serve the blueberry oatmeal muffins as a delicious breakfast or snack.

Chocolate Avocado Mousse:

Preparation time: 10 minutes

Chilling time: 2 hours

Servings: 4

Ingredients:

- 2 ripe avocados

- 1/4 cup of unsweetened cocoa powder

- 1/4 cup of maple syrup or agave nectar

- 1/4 cup of almond milk (or any other milk of your choice)

- 1 teaspoon of vanilla extract

- Pinch of salt

- Optional toppings: whipped cream, shaved chocolate, berries

Directions:

1. Cut the avocados in half, remove the pits, and scoop out the flesh.

2. Place the avocado flesh, cocoa powder, maple syrup or agave nectar, almond milk, vanilla extract, and salt in a blender or food processor.

3. Blend until smooth and creamy, scraping down the sides as needed.

4. Taste and adjust the sweetness if desired, adding more maple syrup or agave nectar.

5. Transfer the mousse to individual serving cups or bowls.

6. Cover and refrigerate for at least 2 hours to allow the mousse to set.

7. Optional: Before serving, top the chocolate avocado mousse with whipped cream, shaved chocolate, or berries for added flavor and decoration.

8. Serve the mousse chilled as a satisfying and healthier dessert option.

APPLE CINNAMON CRUMBLE BARS:

Preparation time: 15 minutes

Baking time: 30-35 minutes

Servings: 12

Ingredients:

- 2 cups of all-purpose flour

- 1I apologize for the inconvenience, but it seems that the response got cut off after providing the ingredients for the Apple Cinnamon Crumble Bars. Here's the complete recipe:

Apple Cinnamon Crumble Bars:

Preparation time: 15 minutes

Baking time: 30-35 minutes

Servings: 12

Ingredients:

- 2 cups of all-purpose flour

- 1 cup of rolled oats

- 1 cup of packed brown sugar

- 1/2 teaspoon of baking soda

- 1/2 teaspoon of salt

- 1 teaspoon of ground cinnamon

- 3/4 cup of unsalted butter, melted

- 2 cups of peeled, cored, and diced apples

- 2 tablespoons of granulated sugar

- 1 tablespoon of all-purpose flour

- 1/2 teaspoon of ground cinnamon

- 1/4 teaspoon of ground nutmeg

Directions:

1. Preheat your oven to 350°F (175°C). Grease a 9x13-inch baking pan.

2. In a large bowl, combine the flour, rolled oats, brown sugar, baking soda, salt, and ground cinnamon.

3. Pour in the melted butter and stir until the mixture resembles coarse crumbs.

4. Set aside 1 1/2 cups of the crumb mixture for the topping.

5. Press the remaining crumb mixture evenly into the bottom of the prepared baking pan.

6. In a separate bowl, combine the diced apples, granulated sugar, flour, ground cinnamon, and ground nutmeg. Toss until the apples are coated.

7. Spread the apple mixture evenly over the crust in the baking pan.

8. Sprinkle the reserved crumb mixture over the top of the apples.

9. Bake in the preheated oven for 30-35 minutes, or until the top is golden brown and the apples are tender.

10. Remove from the oven and let it cool completely in the pan on a wire rack.

11. Once cooled, cut into bars and serve as a delightful treat.

CARROT CAKE WITH CREAM CHEESE FROSTING:

Preparation time: 30 minutes

Baking time: 30-35 minutes

Servings: 12

Ingredients:

For the cake:

- 2 cups of all-purpose flour

- 2 teaspoons of baking powder

- 1 1/2 teaspoons of baking soda

- 1/2 teaspoon of salt

- 1 1/2 teaspoons of ground cinnamon

- 1/2 teaspoon of ground nutmeg

- 1/2 cup of vegetable oil

- 1 cup of granulated sugar

- 1 cup of packed brown sugar

- 4 large eggs

- 2 teaspoons of vanilla extract

- 3 cups of grated carrots

- 1 cup of crushed pineapple, drained

- 1/2 cup of chopped walnuts or pecans (optional)

For the cream cheese frosting:

- 8 ounces of cream cheese, softened

- 1/2 cup of unsalted butter, softened

- 4 cups of powdered sugar

- 1 teaspoon of vanilla extract

Directions:

1. Preheat your oven to 350°F (175°C). Grease and flour a 9x13-inch baking pan or two 9-inch round cake pans.

2. In a large bowl, whisk together the flour, baking powder, baking soda, salt, cinnamon, and nutmeg.

3. In a separate bowl, whisk together the vegetable oil, granulated sugar, brown sugar, eggs, and vanilla extract until well combined.

4. Pour the wet ingredients into the dry ingredients and mix until just combined.

5. Fold in the grated carrots, crushed pineapple, and chopped walnuts or pecans (if using).

6. Pour the batter into the prepared baking pan(s) and spread it evenly.

7. Bake in the preheated oven for 30-35 minutes, or until a toothpick inserted into the center comes out clean.

8. Remove from the oven and let the cake cool completely in the pan(s) on a wire rack.

9. In the meantime, prepare the cream cheese frosting. In a bowl, beat the softened cream cheese and butter until smooth and creamy.

10. Gradually add the powdered sugar, one cup at a time, beating well after each addition.

11. Stir in the vanilla extract and continue beating until the frosting is light and fluffy.

12. Once the cake has cooled, frost it with the cream cheese frosting.

13. Slice and serve the carrot cake with cream cheese frosting as a delightful dessert.

Lemon Poppy Seed Loaf:

Preparation time: 15 minutes

Baking time: 45-50 minutes

Servings: 8-10

Ingredients:

- 1 1/2 cups of all-purpose flour

- 2 tablespoons of poppy seeds

- 1 teaspoon of baking powder

- 1/2 teaspoon of baking soda

- 1/4 teaspoon of salt

- 1/2 cup of unsalted butter, softened

- 1 cup of granulated sugar

- 2 large eggs

- 1 teaspoon of vanilla extract

- 1 tablespoon of lemon zest

- 1/4 cup of fresh lemon juice

- 1/2 cup of buttermilk

For the lemon glaze:

- 1 cup of powdered sugar

- 2 tablespoons of fresh lemon juice

Directions:

1. Preheat your oven to 350°F (175°C). Grease and flour a 9x5-inch loaf pan.

2. In a medium bowl, whisk together the flour, poppy seeds, baking powder, baking soda, and salt. Set aside.

3. In a large bowl, cream together the softened butter and granulated sugar until light and fluffy.

4. Add the eggs, one at a time, beating well after each addition. Stir in the vanilla extract, lemon zest, and lemon juice.

5. Gradually add the dry ingredients to the wet ingredients, alternating with buttermilk. Begin and end with the dry ingredients, mixing until just combined.

6. Pour the batter into the prepared loaf pan and smooth the top with a spatula.

7. Bake in the preheated oven for 45-50 minutes, or until a toothpick inserted into the center comes out clean.

8. While the loaf is still warm, prepare the lemon glaze. In a small bowl, whisk together the powdered sugar and lemon juice until smooth.

9. Once the loaf has cooled for about 10 minutes, remove it from the pan and place it on a wire rack. Drizzle the lemon glaze over the top.

10. Let the loaf cool completely before slicing and serving.

PEANUT BUTTER CHOCOLATE CHIP COOKIES:

Preparation time: 15 minutes

Baking time: 10-12 minutes

Servings: 24 cookies

Ingredients:

- 1 1/4 cups of all-purpose flour

- 1/2 teaspoon of baking soda

- 1/4 teaspoon of salt

- 1/2 cup of unsalted butter, softened

- 1/2 cup of creamy peanut butter

- 1/2 cup of granulated sugar

- 1/2 cup of packed brown sugar

- 1 large egg

- 1 teaspoon of vanilla extract

- 1 cup of semi-sweet chocolate chips

Directions:

1. Preheat your oven to 375°F (190°C). Line a baking sheet with parchment paper.

2. In a medium bowl, whisk together the flour, baking soda, and salt. Set aside.

3. In a large bowl, cream together the softened butter, peanut butter, granulated sugar, and brown sugar until light and fluffy.

4. Add the egg and vanilla extract to the butter mixture and mix well.

5. Gradually add the dry ingredients to the wet ingredients, mixing until just combined.

6. Stir in the chocolate chips until evenly distributed throughout the dough.

7. Drop rounded tablespoons of dough onto the prepared baking sheet, spacing them about 2 inches apart.

8. Bake in the preheated oven for 10-12 minutes, or until the edges are golden brown.

9. Remove from the oven and let the cookies cool on the baking sheet for a few minutes before transferring them to a wire rack to cool completely.

10. Enjoy the delicious peanut butter chocolate chip cookies with a glass of cold milk.

ZUCCHINI BREAD WITH DARK CHOCOLATE CHIPS:

Preparation time: 15 minutes

Baking time: 50-60 minutes

Servings: 8-10

Ingredients:

- 2 cups of all-purpose flour

- 1 teaspoon of baking powder

- 1/2 teaspoon of baking soda

- 1/2 teaspoon of salt

- 1 teaspoon of ground cinnamon

- 1/2 teaspoon of ground nutmeg

- 1/2 cup of granulated sugar

- 1/2 cup of packed brown sugar

- 1/2 cup of unsalted butter, melted

- 2 large eggs

- 1 teaspoon of vanilla extract

- 1 1/2 cups of grated zucchini

- 1 cup of dark chocolate chips

Directions:

1. Preheat your oven to 350°F (175°C). Grease and flour a 9x5-inch loaf pan.

2. In a medium bowl, whisk together the flour, baking powder, baking soda, salt, cinnamon, and nutmeg. Set aside.

3. In a large bowl, combine the granulated sugar, brown sugar, melted butter, eggs, and vanilla extract. Mix well.

4. Gradually add the dry ingredients to the wet ingredients, mixing until just combined.

5. Fold in the grated zucchini and dark chocolate chips until evenly distributed throughout the batter.

6. Pour the batter into the prepared loaf pan and smooth the top with a spatula.

7. Bake in the preheated oven for 50-60 minutes, or until a toothpick inserted into the center comes out clean.

8. Allow the zucchini bread to cool in the pan for about 10 minutes, then transfer it to a wire rack to cool completely before slicing and serving.

RASPBERRY ALMOND THUMBPRINT COOKIES:

Preparation time: 20 minutes

Baking time: 12-15 minutes

Servings: 24 cookies

Ingredients:

- 1 cup of unsalted butter, softened

- 2/3 cup of granulated sugar

- 1/2 teaspoon of almond extract

- 2 cups of all-purpose flour

- 1/2 cup of seedless raspberry jam

For the glaze:

- 1 cup of powdered sugar

- 2-3 tablespoons of milk

- 1/2 teaspoon of almond extract

Directions:

1. Preheat your oven to 350°F (175°C). Line a baking sheet with parchment paper.

2. In a large bowl, cream together the softened butter, granulated sugar, and almond extract until light and fluffy.

3. Gradually add the flour to the butter mixture, mixing until the dough comes together.

4. Roll the dough into 1-inch balls and place them on the prepared baking sheet, spacing them about 2 inches apart.

5. Use your thumb or the back of a spoon to make an indentation in the center of each cookie.

6. Fill each indentation with about 1/2 teaspoon of raspberry jam.

7. Bake in the preheated oven for 12-15 minutes, or until the edges of the cookies are lightly golden.

8. Remove from the oven and let the cookies cool on the baking sheet for a few minutes before transferring them to a wire rack to cool completely.

9. In a small bowl, whisk together the powdered sugar, milk, and almond extract to make the glaze.

10. Drizzle the glaze over the cooled cookies.

11. Allow the glaze to set before serving.

CHOCOLATE CHIP COCONUT BLONDIES:

Preparation time: 15 minutes

Baking time: 25-30 minutes

Servings: 16 blondies

Ingredients:

- 1 cup of all-purpose flour

- 1/2 teaspoon of baking powder

- 1/4 teaspoon of salt

- 1/2 cup of unsalted butter, melted

- 1 cup of packed brown sugar

- 1 large egg

- 1 teaspoon of vanilla extract

- 1/2 cup of shredded coconut

- 1/2 cup of semi-sweet chocolate chips

Directions:

1. Preheat your oven to 350°F (175°C). Grease and flour an 8x8-inch baking pan.

2. In a medium bowl, whisk together the flour, baking powder, and salt. Set aside.

3. In a large bowl, combine the melted butter and brown sugar. Mix well.

4. Add the egg and vanilla extract to the butter mixture and mix until smooth.

5. Gradually add the dry ingredients to the wet ingredients, mixing until just combined.

6. Fold in the shredded coconut and chocolate chips until evenly distributed throughout the batter.

7. Spread the batter evenly into the prepared baking pan.

8. Bake in the preheated oven for 25-30 minutes, or until a toothpick inserted into the center comes out with a few moist crumbs.

9. Allow the blondies to cool in the pan before cutting them into squares and serving.

Enjoy these delicious baked treats

STRAWBERRY SHORTCAKE:

Preparation time: 20 minutes

Baking time: 12-15 minutes

Assembly time: 10 minutes

Servings: 4

Ingredients:

- 2 cups of fresh strawberries, hulled and sliced

- 2 tablespoons of granulated sugar

- 2 cups of all-purpose flour

- 1/4 cup of granulated sugar

- 1 tablespoon of baking powder

- 1/2 teaspoon of salt

- 1/2 cup of unsalted butter, cold and cut into small pieces

- 2/3 cup of milk

- Whipped cream or whipped topping for serving

Directions:

1. In a bowl, combine the sliced strawberries and 2 tablespoons of granulated sugar. Toss well and let them sit for about 15 minutes to allow the strawberries to release their juices.

2. Preheat your oven to 425°F (220°C).

3. In a large bowl, whisk together the flour, 1/4 cup of granulated sugar, baking powder, and salt.

4. Add the cold butter pieces to the flour mixture and use a pastry cutter or your fingers to cut the butter into the flour until it resembles coarse crumbs.

5. Pour in the milk and stir until the dough comes together.

6. Turn the dough out onto a lightly floured surface and gently knead it a few times until it holds together.

7. Roll out the dough to a thickness of about 1/2 inch and cut it into rounds using a biscuit cutter.

8. Place the rounds onto a baking sheet and bake in the preheated oven for 12-15 minutes, or until they are golden brown.

9. Remove the shortcakes from the oven and let them cool slightly.

10. To assemble, split the shortcakes in half horizontally. Place the bottom half on a plate, spoon some of the macerated strawberries onto it, and top with a dollop of whipped cream or whipped topping. Place the top half of the shortcake on top and garnish with more strawberries and whipped cream.

11. Serve the strawberry shortcakes immediately.

Vegan Chocolate Cake:

Preparation time: 20 minutes

Baking time: 30-35 minutes

Servings: 8-10

Ingredients:

- 1 1/2 cups of all-purpose flour

- 1 cup of granulated sugar

- 1/4 cup of unsweetened cocoa powder

- 1 teaspoon of baking soda

- 1/2 teaspoon of salt

- 1 cup of almond milk (or any non-dairy milk)

- 1/3 cup of vegetable oil

- 1 tablespoon of apple cider vinegar

- 1 teaspoon of vanilla extract

For the chocolate ganache:

- 1/2 cup of dairy-free chocolate chips

- 1/4 cup of almond milk (or any non-dairy milk)

Directions:

1. Preheat your oven to 350°F (175°C). Grease and flour a 9-inch round cake pan.

2. In a large bowl, whisk together the flour, sugar, cocoa powder, baking soda, and salt.

3. In a separate bowl, whisk together the almond milk, vegetable oil, apple cider vinegar, and vanilla extract.

4. Pour the wet ingredients into the dry ingredients and whisk until the batter is smooth and well combined.

5. Pour the batter into the prepared cake pan and smooth the top with a spatula.

6. Bake in the preheated oven for 30-35 minutes, or until a toothpick inserted into the center comes out clean.

7. Remove the cake from the oven and let it cool in the pan for about 10 minutes before transferring it to a wire rack to cool completely.

8. To make the chocolate ganache, combine the chocolate chips and almond milk in a microwave-safe bowl. Microwave in 30-second intervals, stirring well after each interval, until the chocolate is melted and the mixture is smooth.

9. Once the cake has cooled, pour the chocolate ganache over the top, allowing it to drip down the sides.

10. Let the ganache set before serving the vegan chocolate cake.

PUMPKIN SPICE MUFFINS:

Preparation time: 15 minutes

Baking time: 20-25 minutes

Servings: 12 muffins

Ingredients:

- 2 cups of all-purpose flour

- 1 cup of granulated sugar

- 2 teaspoons of baking powder

- 1/2 teaspoon of baking soda

- 1/2 teaspoon of salt

- 2 teaspoons of pumpkin pie spice

- 1 cup of canned pumpkin puree

- 1/2 cup of vegetable oil

- 2 large eggs

- 1 teaspoon of vanilla extract

For the streusel topping:

- 1/4 cup of all-purpose flour

- 1/4 cup of granulated sugar

- 2 tablespoons of unsalted butter, cold and cutinto small pieces

- 1/2 teaspoon of pumpkin pie spice

Directions:

1. Preheat your oven to 375°F (190°C). Line a muffin tin with paper liners or grease the cups.

2. In a large bowl, whisk together the flour, sugar, baking powder, baking soda, salt, and pumpkin pie spice.

3. In a separate bowl, whisk together the pumpkin puree, vegetable oil, eggs, and vanilla extract until well combined.

4. Pour the wet ingredients into the dry ingredients and stir until just combined. Be careful not to overmix.

5. In a small bowl, combine the flour, sugar, butter, and pumpkin pie spice for the streusel topping. Use your fingers or a fork to cut the butter into the dry ingredients until it resembles coarse crumbs.

6. Divide the muffin batter evenly among the prepared muffin cups, filling each about 2/3 full.

7. Sprinkle the streusel topping over the muffin batter, pressing it gently into the surface.

8. Bake in the preheated oven for 20-25 minutes, or until a toothpick inserted into the center of a muffin comes out clean.

9. Remove the muffins from the oven and let them cool in the pan for a few minutes before transferring them to a wire rack to cool completely.

10. Enjoy the pumpkin spice muffins as a delicious fall treat!

Almond Butter Energy Balls:

Preparation time: 15 minutes

Chilling time: 30 minutes

Servings: 12 energy balls

Ingredients:

- 1 cup of rolled oats

- 1/2 cup of almond butter

- 1/4 cup of honey or maple syrup (for a vegan option)

- 1/4 cup of ground flaxseed

- 1/4 cup of mini chocolate chips

- 1/4 cup of chopped nuts (such as almonds or walnuts)

- 1 teaspoon of vanilla extract

- A pinch of salt

Directions:

1. In a large bowl, combine the rolled oats, almond butter, honey or maple syrup, ground flaxseed, chocolate chips, chopped nuts, vanilla extract, and salt.

2. Stir well until all the ingredients are thoroughly combined.

3. Place the mixture in the refrigerator for about 30 minutes to allow it to firm up.

4. After chilling, remove the mixture from the refrigerator and shape it into 1-inch balls using your hands.

5. Store the almond butter energy balls in an airtight container in the refrigerator for up to 1 week.

6. These energy balls make a great snack or quick pick-me-up during the day.

Oatmeal Raisin Cookies:

Preparation time: 15 minutes

Baking time: 10-12 minutes

Servings: Approximately 24 cookies

Ingredients:

- 1 cup of unsalted butter, softened

- 1 cup of packed brown sugar

- 1/2 cup of granulated sugar

- 2 large eggs

- 1 teaspoon of vanilla extract

- 1 1/2 cups of all-purpose flour

- 1 teaspoon of baking soda

- 1 teaspoon of ground cinnamon

- 1/2 teaspoon of salt

- 3 cups of old-fashioned oats

- 1 cup of raisins

Directions:

1. Preheat your oven to 350°F (175°C). Line a baking sheet with parchment paper.

2. In a large bowl, cream together the softened butter, brown sugar, and granulated sugar until light and fluffy.

3. Beat in the eggs, one at a time, and then stir in the vanilla extract.

4. In a separate bowl, whisk together the flour, baking soda, ground cinnamon, and salt.

5. Gradually add the dry ingredients to the butter and sugar mixture, mixing well after each addition.

6. Stir in the oats and raisins until evenly distributed throughout the dough.

7. Drop rounded tablespoons of dough onto the prepared baking sheet, spacing them about 2 inches apart.

8. Bake in the preheated oven for 10-12 minutes, or until the edges are golden brown.

9. Remove the cookies from the oven and let them cool on the baking sheet for a few minutes before transferring them to a wire rack to cool completely.

10. Enjoy the delicious oatmeal raisin cookies with a tall glass of milk or your favorite hot beverage.

BERRY CRISP WITH OAT TOPPING:

Preparation time: 15 minutes

Baking time: 30-35 minutes

Servings: 6

Ingredients:

- 4 cups of mixed berries (such as blueberries, raspberries, and blackberries)

- 1/4 cup of granulated sugar

- 1 tablespoon of cornstarch

- 1 tablespoon of lemon juice

- 1 cup of old-fashioned oats

- 1/2 cup of all-purpose flour

- 1/2 cup of packed brown sugar

- 1/2 teaspoon of ground cinnamon

- 1/4 teaspoon of salt

- 1/2 cup of unsalted butter, melted

Directions:

1. Preheat your oven to 375°F (190°C). Grease a 9-inch baking dish.

2. In a large bowl, combine the mixed berries, granulated sugar, cornstarch, and lemon juice. Toss well to coat the berries evenly.

3. In a separate bowl, mix together the oats, flour, brown sugar, cinnamon, and salt.

4. Pour the melted butter over the oat mixture and stir until the ingredients are well combined and crumbly.

5. Spread the berry mixture evenly in the greased baking dish.

6. Sprinkle the oat topping over the berries, covering them completely.

7. Bake in the preheated oven for 30-35 minutes, or until the topping is golden brown and the berries are bubbling.

8. Remove the berry crisp from the oven and let it cool for a few minutes before serving.

9. Serve the warm berry crisp with a scoop of vanilla ice cream or a dollop of whipped cream, if desired.

CHOCOLATE PEANUT BUTTER CUPS:

Preparation time: 30 minutes

Chilling time: 1 hour

Servings: Approximately 12 peanut butter cups

Ingredients:

- 12 ounces of semisweet or dark chocolate, chopped

- 1/2 cup of creamy peanut butter

- 1/4 cup of powdered sugar

- 1/4 teaspoon of salt

Directions:

1. Line a muffin tin with paper liners.

2. In a microwave-safe bowl, melt half of the chopped chocolate in the microwave in 30-second intervals, stirring well after each interval, until it is completely melted and smooth.

3. Spoon about 1 tablespoon of melted chocolate into each paper liner, spreading it evenly along the bottom and slightly up the sides.

4. Place the muffin tin in the refrigerator or freezer to allow the chocolate to set.

5. In a separate bowl, mix together the peanut butter, powdered sugar, and salt until well combined.

6. Remove the muffin tin from the refrigerator or freezer and spoon about 1 teaspoon of the peanut butter mixture into each chocolate-lined cup.

7. Flatten the peanut butter mixture slightly with the back of a spoon.

8. Melt the remaining chopped chocolate in the microwave using the same method as before.

9. Spoon another tablespoon of melted chocolate over the peanut butter mixture in each cup, making sure to cover the peanut butter completely.

10. Gently tap the muffin tin on the counter to even out the chocolate and remove any air bubbles.

11. Return the muffin tin to the refrigerator or freezer and chill until the chocolate is firm, about 1 hour.

12. Once the chocolate peanut butter cups are completely set, remove them from the paper liners and store in an airtight container in the refrigerator.

Lemon Blueberry Scones:

Preparation time: 15 minutes

Baking time: 18-20 minutes

Servings: 8 scones

Ingredients:

- 2 cups of all-purpose flour

- 1/2 cup of granulated sugar

- 2 teaspoons of baking powder

- 1/2 teaspoon of baking soda

- 1/2 teaspoon of salt

- Zest of 1 lemon

- 1/2 cup of unsalted butter, cold and cut into small pieces

- 1/2 cup of buttermilk

- 1 tablespoon of lemon juice

- 1 cup of fresh or frozen blueberries

- 1 tablespoon of coarse sugar (optional, for sprinkling on top)

For the glaze:

- 1 cup of powdered sugar

- 2 tablespoons of fresh lemon juice

Directions:

1. Preheat your oven to 400°F (200°C). Line a baking sheet with parchment paper.

2. In a large bowl, whisk together the flour, granulated sugar, baking powder, baking soda, salt, and lemon zest.

3. Add the cold butter pieces to the flour mixture and use a pastry cutter or your fingers to cut the butter into the flour until it resembles coarse crumbs.

4. In a separate bowl, combine the buttermilk and lemon juice. Pour the mixture into the flour mixture and stir until just combined.

5. Gently fold in the blueberries, being careful not to overmix and crush theberries.

6. Turn the dough out onto a lightly floured surface and knead it a few times until it comes together.

7. Pat the dough into a circle about 1 inch thick. Use a sharp knife or a biscuit cutter to cut the dough into 8 wedges.

8. Transfer the scones to the prepared baking sheet, spacing them a few inches apart.

9. If desired, sprinkle the tops of the scones with coarse sugar for added crunch.

10. Bake in the preheated oven for 18-20 minutes, or until the scones are golden brown on top.

11. While the scones are baking, prepare the glaze by whisking together the powdered sugar and lemon juice until smooth.

12. Remove the scones from the oven and let them cool for a few minutes. Drizzle the glaze over the slightly warm scones.

13. Serve the lemon blueberry scones warm or at room temperature.

CINNAMON SUGAR DONUTS:

Preparation time: 15 minutes

Cooking time: 15 minutes

Servings: Approximately 12 donuts

Ingredients:

- 2 cups of all-purpose flour

- 1/2 cup of granulated sugar

- 2 teaspoons of baking powder

- 1/2 teaspoon of baking soda

- 1/2 teaspoon of salt

- 1 teaspoon of ground cinnamon

- 1/2 teaspoon of ground nutmeg

- 3/4 cup of buttermilk

- 2 large eggs

- 2 tablespoons of unsalted butter, melted

- Vegetable oil, for frying

For the cinnamon sugar coating:

- 1/2 cup of granulated sugar

- 1 teaspoon of ground cinnamon

Directions:

1. In a large bowl, whisk together the flour, sugar, baking powder, baking soda, salt, cinnamon, and nutmeg.

2. In a separate bowl, whisk together the buttermilk, eggs, and melted butter.

3. Pour the wet ingredients into the dry ingredients and stir until just combined. Be careful not to overmix.

4. Heat vegetable oil in a deep saucepan or Dutch oven to a temperature of 350°F (175°C).

5. Drop spoonfuls of the dough into the hot oil, being careful not to overcrowd the pan. Fry the donuts for about 2-3 minutes per side, or until they are golden brown.

6. Use a slotted spoon to transfer the donuts to a paper towel-lined plate to drain excess oil.

7. In a shallow bowl, mix together the granulated sugar and ground cinnamon for the coating.

8. While the donuts are still warm, roll them in the cinnamon sugar mixture until they are fully coated.

9. Repeat the frying and coating process with the remaining dough.

10. Serve the cinnamon sugar donuts warm.

MIXED BERRY COBBLER:

Preparation time: 15 minutes

Baking time: 45-50 minutes

Servings: 6-8

Ingredients:

- 4 cups of mixed berries (such as strawberries, blueberries, raspberries, and blackberries)

- 1/2 cup of granulated sugar

- 2 tablespoons of cornstarch

- 1 tablespoon of lemon juice

- 1 cup of all-purpose flour

- 1/2 cup of granulated sugar

- 1 teaspoon of baking powder

- 1/2 teaspoon of salt

- 1/2 cup of unsalted butter, cold and cut into small pieces

- 1/4 cup of boiling water

Directions:

1. Preheat your oven to 375°F (190°C). Grease a 9-inch baking dish.

2. In a large bowl, combine the mixed berries, granulated sugar, cornstarch, and lemon juice. Toss well to coat the berries evenly.

3. Pour the berry mixture into the greased baking dish, spreading it out in an even layer.

4. In a separate bowl, whisk together the flour, granulated sugar, baking powder, and salt.

5. Add the cold butter pieces to the flour mixture and use a pastry cutter or your fingers to cut the butter into the flour until it resembles coarse crumbs.

6. Sprinkle the crumbly mixture over the berries in the baking dish.

7. Pour the boiling water evenly over the entire cobbler.

8. Bake in the preheated oven for 45-50 minutes, or until the topping is golden brown and the berries are bubbling.

9. Remove the mixed berry cobbler from the oven and let it cool for a few minutes before serving.

10. Serve the warm cobbler with a scoop of vanilla ice cream or a dollop of whipped cream, if desired.

Enjoy your delicious homemade treats!

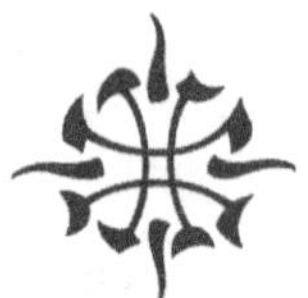

Chapter 7

Tips for a Healthy Lifestyle

INCORPORATING MINDFUL EATING HABITS:

1. Slow down: Take your time to eat and savor each bite. Chew your food thoroughly and pay attention to the taste, texture, and aroma of each bite.

2. Eliminate distractions: Avoid eating in front of the TV or while scrolling on your phone. Instead, create a calm and mindful eating environment by sitting at a table and focusing solely on your meal.

3. Listen to your body: Tune in to your body's hunger and fullness cues. Eat when you're hungry and stop eating when you're comfortably satisfied. Avoid overeating or eating to the point of feeling stuffed.

4. Engage your senses: Pay attention to the colors, smells, and flavors of your food. Eating mindfully involves engaging all of your senses and being fully present in the moment.

5. Practice gratitude: Before you start eating, take a moment to express gratitude for the food on your plate. Recognize the effort and resources that went into providing you with nourishment.

Balancing Macronutrients in Your Diet:

1. Include protein: Protein is essential for building and repairing tissues, as well as for supporting various bodily functions. Include lean sources of protein such as chicken, fish, tofu, beans, and Greek yogurt in your meals.

2. Incorporate healthy fats: Healthy fats are important for brain function, hormone production, and nutrient absorption. Include sources of healthy fats like avocados, nuts, seeds, olive oil, and fatty fish (such as salmon) in your diet.

3. Choose complex carbohydrates: Complex carbohydrates provide sustained energy and are rich in fiber, vitamins, and minerals. Opt for whole grains, legumes, fruits, and vegetables instead of refined and processed carbohydrates.

4. Prioritize vegetables and fruits: These should be the foundation of your meals, providing a wide range of nutrients, fiber, and antioxidants. Aim to fill half of your plate with non-starchy vegetables and include a variety of fruits throughout the day.

5. Practice portion control: Balancing macronutrients also involves portion control. Pay attention to portion sizes and be mindful of your body's hunger and fullness signals to avoid overeating.

THE IMPORTANCE OF HYDRATION:

1. Drink enough water: Aim to drink at least 8 cups (64 ounces) of water per day. However, individual water needs may vary based on factors such as activity level, climate, and overall health.

2. Carry a water bottle: Keep a reusable water bottle with you throughout the day as a reminder to stay hydrated. Sip water regularly and refill your bottle as needed.

3. Infuse water with flavor: If plain water feels boring, add flavor by infusing it with fruits, herbs, or cucumber slices. This can make hydration more enjoyable and encourage you to drink more water.

4. Limit sugary and caffeinated beverages: Beverages like soda, sweetened juices, and caffeinated drinks can contribute to dehydration. Limit your intake of these beverages and opt for water as your primary source of hydration.

5. Pay attention to thirst cues: Thirst is a signal that your body needs water. Listen to your body and drink water when you

feel thirsty. Additionally, be mindful of signs of dehydration, such as dark urine or feeling fatigued, and increase your water intake accordingly.

GROCERY SHOPPING TIPS FOR BLOOD TYPE A:

1. Emphasize fresh fruits and vegetables: Blood type A individuals tend to thrive on a plant-based diet. Choose a variety of fresh, organic fruits and vegetables to provide essential nutrients and antioxidants.

2. Include lean proteins: Opt for lean protein sources such as fish, poultry, tofu, and legumes. These can provide the necessary protein without excessive saturated fats.

3. Prioritize whole grains: Whole grains like quinoa, brown rice, and oats are beneficial for blood type A individuals. They provide complex carbohydrates, fiber, and essential nutrients.

4. Minimize red meat and dairy: Blood type A individuals may have difficulty digesting red meat and dairy products. Consider reducing or eliminating these foods from your diet or opting for alternatives like lean poultry or plant-based milk.

5. Read food labels: Pay attention to food labels to ensure that you're making choices aligned with your blood type recommendations. Look for whole, unprocessed foods and avoid products with additives or artificial ingredients.

Managing Stress for Overall Well-being:

1. Practice relaxation techniques: Engage in activities that promote relaxation, such as deep breathing exercises, meditation, yoga, or tai chi. These practices can help reduce stress and promote a sense of calm.

2. Prioritize self-care: Set aside time for activities that bring you joy and relaxation. This could include hobbies, spending time in nature, taking a bath, or engaging in creative outlets.

3. Exercise regularly: Physical activity is an effective stress reducer. Find an exercise routine that you enjoy, whether it's walking, jogging, dancing, or practicing a sport, and make it a regular part of your routine.

4. Get enough sleep: Lack of sleep can contribute to increasedstress levels. Aim for 7-9 hours of quality sleep each night to support your overall well-being and help manage stress.

5. Seek support: Reach out to friends, family, or a mental health professional for support during stressful times. Talking about your feelings and concerns can provide relief and help you gain different perspectives on managing stress.

6. Practice time management: Prioritize tasks and set realistic goals to avoid feeling overwhelmed. Break larger tasks into smaller, manageable steps and delegate when possible.

7. Limit exposure to stressors: Identify sources of stress in your life and take steps to minimize or avoid them when possible. This could involve setting boundaries, saying no to additional responsibilities, or making lifestyle changes.

8. Incorporate stress-reducing activities: Engage in activities that promote stress reduction, such as listening to calming music, journaling, practicing mindfulness, or engaging in hobbies that bring you joy.

Remember, managing stress is a personal journey, and it's important to find strategies that work best for you. Experiment with different techniques and be patient with yourself as you develop a stress management routine that fits your needs.

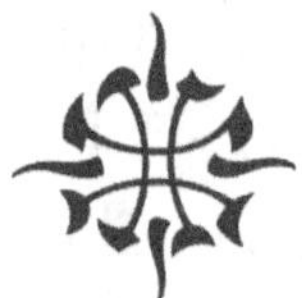

Chapter 8

Conclusion and Beyond

CELEBRATING YOUR JOURNEY WITH BLOOD TYPE A DIET:

1. Acknowledge your progress: Take time to reflect on how far you've come in adopting a blood type A diet. Celebrate the positive changes you've made in your eating habits and the impact it has had on your health and well-being.

2. Reward yourself: Treat yourself to small rewards as you reach milestones or achieve your health goals. It could be something as simple as buying a new cookbook, trying a new recipe, or indulging in a non-food-related treat.

3. Share your success: Share your journey with others who may be interested in the blood type A diet. You can inspire and motivate others by sharing your experiences, recipes, and the positive changes you've experienced.

4. Connect with a community: Join online forums or social media groups focused on the blood type A diet. Engage with others who are following a similar path, exchange ideas, and celebrate your collective progress.

5. Practice self-care: Celebrate your journey by incorporating self-care activities into your routine. This could include taking time for relaxation, pampering yourself, or engaging in activities that bring you joy and fulfillment.

Maintaining a Healthy Vegetarian Lifestyle:

1. Ensure balanced nutrition: As a vegetarian, it's important to include a variety of plant-based proteins, such as legumes, tofu, tempeh, nuts, and seeds, to meet your protein needs. Also, focus on incorporating whole grains, fruits, vegetables, and healthy fats into your diet.

2. Supplement wisely: Pay attention to nutrients that may be lacking in a vegetarian diet, such as vitamin B12, iron, and omega-3 fatty acids. Consider consulting a healthcare professional or registered dietitian to determine if you need any supplements.

3. Experiment with plant-based sources of protein: Explore different sources of plant-based proteins to keep your meals interesting and diverse. Try new recipes with ingredients like lentils, chickpeas, quinoa, edamame, and nutritional yeast.

4. Plan your meals: Planning your meals in advance can help ensure you have a balanced vegetarian diet. Include a variety of colorful fruits and vegetables, whole grains, and plant-based proteins in your meal plan.

5. Stay informed: Keep up-to-date with nutrition information related to vegetarianism. Stay informed about new studies, recipes, and resources that can help you maintain a healthy and sustainable vegetarian lifestyle.

EXPLORING NEW FLAVORS AND INGREDIENTS:

1. Visit ethnic grocery stores: Explore specialty stores that cater to different cuisines. You'll find a wide range of unique ingredients and flavors that can inspire you to try new recipes and expand your culinary horizons.

2. Experiment with spices and herbs: Spices and herbs can transform a dish and add depth of flavor. Try incorporating different spices and herbs into your cooking to create new and exciting taste experiences.

3. Join a cooking class or workshop: Enroll in a cooking class or workshop that focuses on a specific cuisine or cooking technique. This can introduce you to new flavors, ingredients, and cooking methods.

4. Follow food blogs and social media accounts: Discover food blogs and social media accounts that feature recipes and stories from around the world. This can give you inspiration and ideas for trying new flavors and ingredients.

5. Challenge yourself with international recipes: Pick a country or region and explore their traditional recipes. Try recreating dishes from different cultures to broaden your culinary knowledge and palate.

Sharing Your Recipes and Inspiring Others:

1. Start a food blog or social media account: Share your recipes, cooking tips, and experiences on a food blog or social media platform. This allows you to connect with a wider audience and inspire others to explore new flavors and ingredients.

2. Host cooking demonstrations or workshops: Organize cooking demonstrations or workshops in your community or online. Share your favorite recipes, techniques, and insights with others who are interested in learning from you.

3. Participate in recipe exchanges: Join recipe exchange groups or events where you can share your favorite recipes and discover new ones from other food enthusiasts. This fosters a sense of community and encourages culinary exploration.

4. Collaborate with other food enthusiasts: Team up with other food bloggers or individuals passionate about cooking. Collaborate on recipe collections, cookbooks, or joint cooking events to reach a wider audience and share your expertise.

5. Share your story: Personalize your recipes by sharing the stories and inspirations behind them. Connect with your audience on a deeper level by sharing your own journey, challenges, and successes in the kitchen.

CONTINUING YOUR CULINARY ADVENTURE:

1. Keep trying new recipes: Continue to challenge yourself by trying new recipes regularly. Experiment with different cuisines, ingredients, and cooking techniques to keep your culinary journey exciting and fresh.

2. Explore seasonal and local produce: Stay connected to the seasons and explore local farmers' markets or community-supported agriculture (CSA) programs. Experiment with fresh, seasonal produce to create unique and flavorful dishes.

3. Attend food festivals and events: Attend food festivals and events in your area or even travel to experience different culinary traditionsand flavors. Immerse yourself in the vibrant food culture and try dishes from various cuisines.

4. Continue learning: Take cooking classes, attend workshops, or enroll in culinary courses to expand your knowledge and skills. Learn new techniques, discover innovative ingredients, and refine your cooking abilities.

5. Document your culinary adventures: Keep a journal or create a digital record of your culinary adventures. Document your favorite recipes, memorable meals, and unique experiences. This allows you to reflect on your culinary journey and inspire others with your stories.

Remember to enjoy the process and embrace the joy of cooking and discovering new flavors. Your culinary adventure is a continuous exploration, and there's always something new to learn and experience in the world of food.